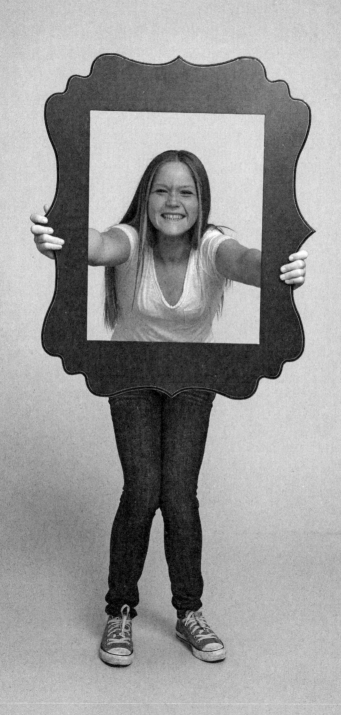

WHO'S THE new KID?

How an ordinary mom helped her
daughter overcome childhood
obesity—*and you can too!*

HEIDI BOND
with JENNA GLATZER

Tyndale House Publishers, Inc.
Carol Stream, Illinois

Visit Tyndale online at www.tyndale.com.

TYNDALE and Tyndale's quill logo are registered trademarks of Tyndale House Publishers, Inc.

Designed by Jacqueline L. Nuñez

Edited by Stephanie Rische

Published in association with the literary agency of William K. Jensen Literary Agency, 119 Bampton Court, Eugene, OR 97404.

Library of Congress Cataloging-in-Publication Data

Bond, Heidi.
   Who's the new kid? : how an ordinary mom helped her daughter overcome childhood obesity, and you can too! / Heidi Bond with Jenna Glatzer.
      pages cm
   Includes bibliographical references.
   ISBN 978-1-4964-0214-1 (hc)
1. Obesity in children.   2. Weight loss.   3. Parent and child.   4. Nutrition.
5. Exercise.   I. Title.
   RJ399.C6B66 2015
   618.92'398—dc23   2014049335

Printed in the United States of America

21	20	19	18	17	16	15
7	6	5	4	3	2	1

I dedicate this book to Breanna and Nathan and all the precious children around the world who are struggling with childhood obesity. I pray you will find comfort in knowing that you are not alone and that there is a heavenly Father who loves you and has a perfect plan for you. I hope that each day of your journey you will find something to be grateful for, whether it's a kind word, a smile from somebody walking by, or an amazing sunset that transforms the sky. I hope you will come to realize that other people's thoughts and opinions of you do not define who you are. You are a child of God, and that is something no one can take away from you. I wish I could be there with you every day of this incredible, life-changing, rewarding journey to share your milestones, joys, pains, and transformations.

Contents

CHAPTER 1

SHE'LL GROW INTO IT

"Mommy! He called me fat!"

My little girl, just on the cusp of three years old, came running over to me at the park with tears streaming down her face.

"Who?" I asked. "Show me who!"

I was filled with mama-bear rage. How dare someone call my daughter names? I took her by the hand, and we walked around until she pointed out the culprit. He was about five years old and didn't *look* like a monster, yet I was amazed at how much anger I could summon against a child. Hadn't his parents taught him not to call other kids names? For goodness' sake, she hadn't even had her third birthday yet! He was picking on a girl who was practically a baby.

I wish I could tell you that I walked right over and had a calm but stern conversation about empathy with the boy and his mother, but the truth is that I don't remember anything after the rage. I just remember wanting to scoop up my little girl and protect her from all the hurts in the world. It was a beautiful day, and we'd been having such a good mother-daughter time at the park. But after that, all I wanted to do was to get her home and make it all better.

"Listen to me," I told Breanna in the car on the way home. "Just because someone says something doesn't make it true. You are beautiful. You're perfect just the way God made you. He doesn't make mistakes."

I said it . . . but even in that moment, I knew her body wasn't "perfect." I knew that my little girl was overweight—and no longer in just a cute "baby fat" way. I'd never imagined something like this would happen to her at such a young age, but something told me that this wouldn't be the last time she'd be called names.

Later that night, I lay in bed reflecting on the day. "Please, God, help us," I called out. "Don't let my sweet daughter be hurt like that ever again. Don't let the cruelty from other people's hearts and words leave any scars."

• • •

Breanna was born in April 2002 at twenty inches long and weighing seven pounds, four ounces. She had big, green-blue eyes, reddish-brown hair, and the softest skin imaginable. She was healthy and happy and beautiful, just as we'd prayed she would be.

I've heard it said that once you have a child, your heart forever walks around in someone else's body. I knew this to be true from the moment I first held my newborn daughter.

I was mesmerized by this person who had just taken her first breaths, and I was surprised to find that motherhood awakened in me both a fierce protectiveness and a consuming love. I knew that I'd move heaven and earth for this little girl.

Things went well for the first year of Breanna's life—she was an easy baby, and we were happy parents. The doctor told me that breastfeeding was best, so that's what I did. She loved feeding times and would get such a contented look on her face after she ate.

"She looks milk-drunk," my husband, Dan, said after she finished.

The way she fed was interesting to us—not leisurely with stops and starts like most babies, but ravenously and quickly. She would drink and drink for ten or fifteen minutes, and then she'd throw her arms back and fall into a deep sleep, as if to say, "Ah, that was just what I needed."

I breastfed her exclusively for about a year before moving her on to solids. I fed her rice cereal and jars of baby food—but only fruits. I bought a couple of jars of vegetables, took one sniff, and thought, *Blech!* I figured a baby surely wouldn't want to eat something that smelled that horrible, so I didn't make her eat any vegetables. I wish I'd realized then how easy it is to blend or mash up real fruits and vegetables for a baby rather than relying on the prepackaged, processed stuff on store shelves.

It wasn't long before Breanna started eating the foods Dan and I ate. She joined us for meals that often included fried chicken, mashed potatoes with lots of butter, cheeseburgers and fries, cheesy enchiladas, white pastas with rich sauces,

Stroganoff, chips, corn dogs, and ice cream, with rare fruits and hardly a vegetable in sight—my own brand of down-home cooking. The litmus test for every meal I made boiled down to one question: Did it taste good? I didn't have any concept of how much salt or fat was in any given meal, nor did I make an effort to include whole grains or fresh produce. I was like a supercharged Paula Deen—if a little butter was good, more was even better!

Our cupboards were stocked with potato chips, Cheetos, and Doritos. I loved fast food (Dan once said he never thought he'd eat McDonald's as an adult until he met me!). I cooked food in butter and Crisco, and I used mayonnaise on my food the way other people use ketchup. Ever since I was a child, I had put mayonnaise on *everything*. When we went to friends' homes for dinner, I would ask my father to bring along a little jar of mayonnaise so I could add it to whatever food might be served. As adults, Dan and I loved having friends over and laying out a big spread of fattening foods.

That was how we ate. It was how we'd always eaten, and we were fine.

Weren't we?

Breanna had a tremendous appetite, which I thought was a blessing at first. She was not one of those picky eaters who had to be coaxed into taking every bite. My girl loved every-thing I made and just wanted more, more, more. It was fun to feed her new foods and watch her light up with pleasure when she tried different tastes and textures for the first time.

As for me, I loved cooking for my family. I had an endless supply of delicious recipes to make and serve. I had no idea if they were nutritious; that notion didn't even register with me. Family dinners were big affairs with plenty of meats and side dishes—and dessert. Of course, dessert. Dan's mom's delicacies were particular favorites. She's a world-class baker, and she always made cakes, breads, and pastries for the family. To me, those cheesecake bars, toffee, fresh apple pies, and Rocky Road cookies—recipes that had been handed down from generation to generation—were a form of love.

I, too, wanted to show my love to my husband and daughter by making them food.

The problem was that both of them had weight struggles. Dan and his brother were opposite body types: they could eat exactly the same thing, and Dan would gain weight while his brother would stay thin. Too thin, even. My husband, on the other hand, struggled to keep at a healthy weight for his six-foot-three frame.

Before I met Dan, I didn't know about the complications of yo-yo dieting. He'd managed to lose the extra weight a few times, but then he'd put it back on. As a result, he needed to have his gallbladder removed. I learned that this isn't uncommon—when people are overweight and lose weight too quickly (more than three pounds per week), they're at an increased risk for gallstones—solid crystals of digestive fluid in the gallbladder that can be as small as a grain of sand or up to the size of a golf ball. Most gallstones are asymptomatic, but sometimes they cause terrible pain, nausea, vomiting, and infection, which is when surgeons have to step in.

Dan had other physical side effects due to weight problems, but the emotional scars were worse. As a kid, he had endured a lot of bullying because of his size, and to this day, those are still some of his most vivid memories. That's exactly what I feared for Breanna.

She obviously inherited his metabolism, I thought.

She was morphing from a baby everyone described as "the cutest baby I've ever seen" to a toddler who elicited reactions like, "Wow, she sure is a big girl."

I knew it was true. I knew it, but I didn't know what to do about it. When we'd gone for her two-year-old checkup with the pediatrician, I went in with my tail between my legs, waiting for a lecture about what I was doing wrong. The doctor and I went over her milestones—she was hitting all of them right on schedule—and then talked about her overall health.

"I know she's overweight," I said.

"She's fine," the doctor said. "Look here." He showed me a growth chart that displayed the average trajectory of a child's height and weight. "She's over the 100th percentile for weight, but she's also over the 100th percentile for height. You don't need to worry. She looks heavy now, but she'll grow into it."

Oh.

Well, that was reassuring. I was not altogether sure that the fat rolls I was seeing bunching up in unexpected places were okay, but this man was a well-regarded pediatrician, and he'd been dealing with children for a long time. I figured he would tell me if there was something that needed to change, so I just forged ahead as I'd been doing. I continued to feed Breanna everything Dan and I ate, and I gave her lollipops and sugary snacks whenever we were out together. After all, she was a kid, and that's what kids like.

For a brief time, I enrolled Breanna in a dance class. She

seemed to enjoy it, and I got a kick out of watching her point her toes and twirl around with a class full of adorable girls. It didn't escape me, though, that Breanna seemed much heavier than the rest of the class.

She'll grow into it, I reminded myself. *The doctor said so.*

But almost a year later, she wasn't growing into it. If anything, the problem was getting worse. And then I got pregnant again. If there was a tipping point, that was it.

• • •

At three years old, Breanna could have kept up with dance class and started eating healthier and maybe slimmed down. But what happened instead was that I got miserably sick right from the beginning of my pregnancy, and Breanna was just about on her own.

I was so ill that I pretty much spent the first five months of my pregnancy shuffling from the bed to the bathroom. I was not only physically sick but also an emotional wreck. Up until that point, I had loved being a stay-at-home mom and spending time with Breanna. But now I was just about absent from her life.

I'd been just as sick when I was pregnant with Breanna, but I didn't have a child to take care of then. Now I managed to pull myself together enough to get her dressed, make her meals, and give her a bath, but that was about it. I'd microwave something for her and sit her in front of the television in my room, and then I'd go back to bed. That way she was safe and close to me, even if I couldn't be actively involved with her.

Those months were a blur for me. I knew what time it

was based on the television theme songs that played in the background: if I heard *Dora the Explorer*, it must be two o'clock. If I heard, "Whose clues? Blue's clues!" then it must be three o'clock.

There was no more dance class. We didn't go to the park. Breanna didn't even play in the yard. She just sat on the chair in my room, watching TV.

That's when things went from bad to worse for Breanna. It was the perfect storm: a kid who was already overweight and preferred sitting to running around, plus a mom so incapacitated that the three-year-old was left to watch television and eat whatever she wanted out of the cupboards all day. And boy, did she ever. Doritos, cookies, chips—and one day I found that she'd eaten an entire bag of Hawaiian rolls that I was planning to serve with dinner. Twelve rolls! She had no stopping point; she'd just keep eating until someone physically took the food away from her. And then she'd throw a fit.

"Please, Mommy. Please. *Please!* I'm so hungry. Mommy, I'm hungry!"

It was like a cartoon—one that would have been funny if it weren't so frustrating.

"Please, please, *please!*"

"No more, honey. We'll be eating dinner soon. Just watch your show."

"But I'm *so* hungry! Please!"

"You've already had a snack. That's enough."

"But I'm still hungry! Please, I need one more snack. One more, please! Please, Mommy!"

How much of that can a person take? For me, it was about two minutes. Then I'd give in, and everything would be quiet again. When I didn't cave, I could expect the tears to follow. Breanna wasn't rude or bratty, but she was persistent—an unstoppable beggar with a laser-beam focus on food. She would cry for several minutes if she didn't get the food she was asking for, until I was genuinely worried that this child was going to physically suffer if I didn't give her the bag of chips *right now*. My mother's heart believed my child was in need, and I thought I had to respond to that by giving her what she was pleading for.

Dan and I both gave in a lot more often than we should have, but we kept hoping the problem would work itself out as she got older. Maybe she'd learn more self-control as she matured, or maybe we'd find an explanation for her never-ending appetite.

But then we began noticing a disturbing trend whenever Breanna slept: she would periodically stop breathing and then gasp for air.

"What do you think that's about?" I asked Dan.

"We should get it checked out," he agreed.

It was scary to watch. Whenever Breanna would stop breathing, I'd hold my breath too, trying not to panic while I waited for her next breath. Although her breathing was always heavy, those episodes, which seemed to occur several times a night, struck terror in me.

The doctor asked us to record Breanna while she slept so he could hear what was happening. It didn't take long to get what we needed; within about an hour, she had one of her episodes. When we went back to the doctor, his diagnosis shook us. She had sleep apnea.

At three years old?

"We'll need to remove her tonsils and adenoids," the doctor explained.

"You mean surgery?" I asked.

"Yes, but it's pretty routine. Just a one-night stay and then she can recover at home."

"Do we need to do it now?" I asked. "I'm going through a very difficult pregnancy."

"You really should schedule it as soon as possible," he said. "Sleep apnea is a dangerous condition, especially for someone so young."

So a couple of weeks later, Breanna was in her little blue gown in the cold hospital room. As a parent, you always try not to pass your fears on to your children. But it was hard; I was terrified to send my daughter off to be anesthetized and to have a surgeon operate on her. Even worse, we had to sign a paper agreeing that we wouldn't sue the doctor if she died on the table. If she *died*? It wasn't a comforting thought as she headed to the operating room.

The nurses put her in a red wagon in place of a gurney, and we waved at her, forcing big, fake smiles. But as soon as she was out of sight, Dan and I broke down. I'm sure the surgery didn't take long, but every minute your child is in surgery feels like an eternity. The only thing left to do was pray and pace the waiting room.

Please, God, guide the surgeon's hand, Dan and I prayed. *Let her be okay.*

• • •

Dan and I were still new Christians then. I hadn't been raised with faith, except for a summer at a Christian camp where

I accepted Jesus as my Savior, but after getting married and thinking about starting a family, I knew I wanted a spiritual foundation that I hadn't had as a child.

When I got pregnant, I felt an emptiness—a yearning for something more. I didn't know exactly what it was, but I thought maybe the best place to start was to go to church. Dan didn't really want to "waste" his day off like that, but he went anyway because he loved me.

Later I read a quote by Beth Moore from *Breaking Free* that explained where I was: "The most obvious symptom of a soul in need of God's satisfaction is a sense of inner emptiness. The awareness of a 'hollow place' somewhere deep inside."

I wanted to experience the kind of community I'd heard about from people who attended church. *A church family*, I thought. *That's what we need.* My original thought was that this would be for Breanna—that she would develop a moral grounding and have something to believe in. But the more we learned each week, the more God pulled on our heartstrings. I wasn't just going for my child's sake anymore, and Dan wasn't just going for me. The truth of Scripture resonated in our souls, encouraging us to wholeheartedly adopt God's ways as our own. As an unexpected benefit, Dan and I were growing in our marriage. We'd always had a solid relationship, but now it was stronger.

Dan joined men's groups at church, and I joined women's Bible studies and volunteered in various ministries. To our delight, we found a family in our church community—like-minded people who wanted to grow spiritually and raise their children to know and love God. Our pastor frequently came over for dinner, and it was at the dinner table where my husband accepted Jesus

Christ as his Lord and Savior. Shortly after Breanna was born, when I was twenty-nine, Dan and I were baptized together.

We learned that we liked God's way a lot more than we liked our own way, and having a baby made us feel profoundly thankful to our Creator. We believed that she was made in his image and that although she had been entrusted to us, she was truly his child—precious and valuable in his sight. And now, as she was behind closed doors in a surgical room, she was in his hands. It was the first time my faith had to face a real test. My daughter was facing a critical moment, and I was powerless to do anything but remain in constant prayer.

I was feeling especially sick on the day of the surgery, and the stress was not helping my nausea one bit. Finally, just as it felt like I would burst into pieces without some kind of news, a nurse came into the waiting area.

"All finished!" she said. "It went fine. She's crying for you in the recovery area, but you can't go in there yet. We'll let you know when it's time."

It was all I could do not to bolt right past the nurse and burst into the recovery room. How could I stay put when I knew my little girl was hurting? I had no idea if there were any nurses or doctors soothing her, but even if so, she didn't know them. She needed *us*.

At last we were allowed to see her as they pushed her gurney to the elevator, ready to go to her room. The moment she saw us, she threw her arms out. "Mommy!"

That's when I knew how scared she was. Typically Breanna is Daddy's girl. She doesn't run for me; she goes straight to him. So the fact that she flung herself at me told me she was desperate to be comforted by whoever she saw first. My heart broke for her, and as soon as she was in the room, I crawled into bed next to her. A few minutes later, though, I had to get up, tripping over her IV lines as I made my way to the bathroom to throw up. Morning sickness has no sense of decorum.

"Maybe they should admit me, too," I told Dan with a wry smile. Too bad it was a children's hospital.

Breanna's recovery involved a lot of Popsicles and rest. In fact, it didn't look a whole lot different from our regular routine at the time, since I was still basically confined to bed, and she watched TV all day anyway.

A typical day for us went something like this: she'd watch *Monsters, Inc.* for the eighty-fifth time, until I had all the words memorized even in my half-asleep state, and when she got hungry, she'd make her way to the pantry or refrigerator. I had no strength to argue. She helped herself to juice, ice cream—whatever she wanted. I was just grateful she was able to swallow and thought it would help her recover faster.

When I was feeling up to it, I wrote letters to Breanna, for her future self to read one day. I'll never forget one of the letters I wrote around that time.

You are three years and six months old now. . . .
I feel scared sometimes when I think about having
to send you to school, because I know how cruel this
world can be. . . . You are now forty-one inches tall
and weigh fifty-two and a half pounds.

Most three-year-old girls weigh twenty-five to thirty-eight pounds. Already, my little girl was clinically obese. By some definitions, she was morbidly obese. This was terrifying territory, because it meant that her life might be cut short because of her weight.

. . .

Breanna was four when Nathan was born in May 2006, and she was thrilled to be a big sister. I loved seeing the two of them together. In the same way that I was protective of Breanna, she was protective of her little brother. She felt a special bond with him from the first time she saw him in the maternity ward.

"If anyone ever hurts you, Brother, I will punch them," she said with all the seriousness of a four-year-old. And really, how could I argue with that? So violent, yet so sweet.

Nathan was six pounds, eight ounces, and 19.5 inches long, with hardly any hair. We all declared him the cutest little boy we'd ever seen. I felt like myself again as soon as he was born, but of course I was consumed with the around-the-clock care a baby needs.

One day, not long after we'd come home from the hospital, I took a good, hard look at my little daughter's ever-growing body and knew I had to do something to make up for all those months of inactivity. The fat rolls were multiplying. Now they were bunching up around her wrists, her knees, and her feet. It was difficult to shop for clothes for her because the regular sizes didn't fit, and she developed sensitivities to fabric where it chafed against her skin.

We signed Breanna up for T-ball, thinking it would be a good way for her to get some exercise. But T-ball, it turns out, is not all that active. It involves a lot of standing around, followed by very short bursts of jogging for twenty feet. She also played soccer at preschool. Dan and I watched as she ran around the field, and we cheered her on. But she pooped out after just a few minutes while the other kids were just getting started.

"Get in there!" I'd yell. "Get the ball! Go! Kick it!"

Dan encouraged her too. "Go, Bre! Look, the ball's right there! Go for it!"

Afterward the parents would give out juice boxes and sugary snacks. That was easily Breanna's favorite part.

I worried as the numbers on the scale rose, and I no longer believed the doctor when he told me that Breanna would "grow into it." She would have to be a giant to accommodate an appetite like hers. By the time she entered kindergarten, she weighed ninety pounds—more than twice what most of her peers weighed—but the pediatrician still waved off my concerns.

"Is there some kind of diet pill she can take to curb her appetite?" I asked.

"No, don't be silly," he said. "She's fine. She's too young for you to worry about this."

"I just feel like something is wrong. She's hungry all the time."

"She's a growing girl," he countered.

"But couldn't it be a thyroid problem or something?"

"No. She's fine."

It was hard to argue. Aside from occasional sore throats, Breanna was rarely sick. And thankfully the surgery had cured the sleep apnea, so she seemed to be healthy. Still, the doctor's words didn't reassure me this time. I was sure there was some underlying medical condition, and I wanted him to send her for tests to find out what was causing this.

I probably could have been sold on just about anything at the time. To me, Breanna was as beautiful as ever, but I worried that it couldn't be healthy for her to weigh double what other kids her age weighed. I was ready for someone to tell me she had a thyroid problem or a hormonal problem or something that was mixing up her brain signals. I wanted a prescription—a quick fix that would make this go away.

TOOLS TO DETERMINE BMI

BMI stands for body mass index. It takes into account height and weight, and it's a reliable indicator of body fat for most kids and teens. Some pediatricians check BMI at annual well-child exams, but here's how to figure it out for yourself:

Step 1: Get an accurate measurement of your child's height.

1. Have your child stand on a hard floor (not carpeted) in bare feet, against a wall or door. He or she should look straight ahead with arms at sides and shoulders level.
2. Use something flat, such as a hardcover book, to place on your child's head at a right angle to the wall or door. The book should rest on the crown of his or her head.
3. Mark the spot where the bottom of the book touches the wall or door. (You can use pencil or chalk and erase it afterward if you want to.)
4. Using a measuring tape, measure from the floor to the mark to the nearest .1 centimeter or 1/8 inch.

Step 2: Get an accurate calculation of your child's weight.

1. Remove your child's shoes and any heavy clothing.
2. Weigh your child on a digital scale that's resting on a hard surface (again, no carpets).

3. If you want to keep track over time, have your child wear the same type of clothing each time you weigh him or her (for example, a T-shirt and shorts), and do the weigh-in at the same time of day—preferably first thing in the morning.

Step 3: Calculate your child's BMI.

1. Use an online calculator to determine your child's BMI based on these measurements. The CDC has a good one here: http://nccd.cdc.gov/dnpabmi/Calculator.aspx. (Note that adult BMI charts and calculators are not the same as those used for children.)

2. You'll get two results: a BMI number and a percentile. The number tells you what the BMI score is, and the percentile tells you where your child falls in relation to other kids who are the same age. Here's what the percentiles mean:

   - Underweight: less than the 5th percentile

   - Healthy weight: 5th percentile up to the 85th percentile

   - Overweight: 85th to less than the 95th percentile

   - Obese: equal to or greater than the 95th percentile

No matter where your child falls in this chart, it's important to make healthy lifestyle choices. If your child falls into the overweight category, it's time to take steps toward healthier eating and exercise and to continue to monitor your child's weight. If your child falls into the obese category, you should take immediate action toward helping your child lose weight.

CHAPTER 2

BAD HABITS START EARLY

"We need to do something," I said to Dan.

"I know," he agreed.

Then we just sort of stared at each other for a while. Neither of us had any idea what, exactly, we were supposed to do. Our combined knowledge about healthy eating and exercise could fit into a Dixie cup.

"The problem is that she can get into everything," I said. "We need to do a better job of keeping her out of the cabinets."

So Dan put a lock on the pantry—an actual lock, with a key. That was a pain, because I had to track down the key every time I wanted to open the pantry, which was multiple times a day. My next step was to move the salty snacks to the upper cabinets where she couldn't reach them.

Or so I thought.

It's impossible to overestimate the resourcefulness of a determined child. Dan once caught Breanna standing on her little wooden chair, which she'd stacked on top of her wooden table so she could reach into the upper cabinets and get the objects of her desire: Doritos, Cheetos, and crackers. We were shocked by the lengths she would go to for the processed foods she craved. What I didn't know was that her body was never satisfied because she was hungry for the real nutrition she rarely got.

I didn't scold her, because I felt guilty. I ate Doritos and Cheetos too, after all. They were my chips, and I was hiding them from her.

After catching Breanna sneaking into cabinets many times, we finally put magnetic child safety locks on the cabinets.

"What are those for?" she asked.

"Oh, that's to keep your little brother safe," Dan said to spare her feelings.

Nathan wasn't even crawling yet; it would be a year or more before we'd have to worry about him getting into the upper shelves. But we didn't want Breanna to know that anything was off limits to her or that we were hiding things. Any sort of slight like this might make her feel different from us— like we were punishing her—and that was not our intention. The idea was to limit her nonchalantly, without her realizing that she was the only one whose food options were being restricted.

The child safety locks were a pain, but they worked pretty well—until I lost the magnetic key. The locked pantry became too much of an annoyance, and we never got another key for the cabinets, and before long Breanna was sneaking food every time our heads were turned. We needed a new plan.

That's when I came up with a great idea: I'd stash my junk food in the garage. The idea remained great for all of six hours.

"Where are you going, Mommy?" Breanna asked that afternoon.

"I'm just going outside for a minute. I'll be right back."

"Can I come with you?"

"No, wait right here."

"I want to come with you. What are you doing out there?"

"Nothing. Just . . . don't worry about it. Can you watch your little brother for me? What a great big sister you are."

I didn't know how to eat a sandwich without Lay's Sour Cream & Onion potato chips. I'm really not kidding—lunch wouldn't feel complete without them, so I was sneaking out to the garage every afternoon to eat my chips in secrecy. Like the locks, this got old really fast, and Breanna was already on to me. I gave up.

I decided it was fine for her to have some chips at lunch and throughout the day like I did; the problem was portion control. If we could just get her appetite down, I thought, we'd be fine.

"Heidi, we're dealing with a child who has a weight prob-lem," Dan gently said to me one day. "We really need to get the junk food out of the house."

"We just need to find a better way to hide it," I argued. I did not want to give up my chips.

"She's going to find it no matter what. I'm telling you as

a person who has been through this my whole life: that stuff can't be in the house anymore."

Reluctantly, I agreed. I went on a raid and threw away all my beloved chips and crackers, and even my bag of Skittles. *Good-bye, old friends.*

The next time I was in the grocery store, I was genuinely perplexed. What was I supposed to buy? If I couldn't get potato chips, what would I serve as a side dish? I looked and looked, but nothing was appealing. Celery sticks? Give me a break! Nothing could match the perfect mix of salty, sweet, and crunchy like a bag full of processed junk food. And so somehow these taboo items wound up in my cart.

I wish I could tell you this happened only once, but that wouldn't be true. We fell into something of a pattern: I'd throw away all the junk, only to buy it again in two weeks or so when my resolve wore off.

I realize now that I was being selfish. This had nothing to do with Breanna; I wanted the junk food, and I didn't have a weight problem, so I thought I was entitled to it. It didn't seem fair that I'd have to give up my favorite foods just because my daughter had a problem. Besides, I didn't think the chips were the underlying issue. I was sure there was a medical condition that was making her want all the chips in the first place.

• • •

The more I read about thyroid problems, the more hope I had that this could be the answer. Since her pediatrician wouldn't test her, I finally decided to bring Breanna to another family practice doctor. It felt a little like going behind his back, but

I was convinced it needed to be done. At that point, it hadn't occurred to me to switch doctors; I still thought her doctor was well qualified and smart—he just wasn't concerned about this particular issue.

When we went in for our appointment, my hopes were high. "My doctor doesn't want to check her thyroid," I said. "But I really think there might be a problem connected to her weight gain." He sent us for blood tests, and a week later, the results came in: her thyroid was fine. I was disappointed—I'd been sure this was our easy answer. The doctor thought Breanna's problem wasn't a medical one—she just needed more activity.

"You should get her into a dance class," he said.

"A dance class is not going to do it," I said. "Her problem goes deeper than that."

Doesn't anyone see what we're up against here? I thought. *We need answers.*

A friend of ours who had diabetes recommended a nutritionist, and we hired him to come to the house and help us make a plan. He measured Breanna and did a body-fat analysis, and he agreed that she needed to lose weight. Her body fat was more than 30 percent; to qualify as healthy for her age, she'd need to be between 14 and 22 percent.

"I recommend more fruits and vegetables and more exercise," he suggested. "You could build an obstacle course in the backyard. Get her up and moving more."

Getting her moving was a challenge. Still, I decided to try the second doctor's advice.

"Hey, Bre, do you want to take a dance class?"

"No."

"Remember how you liked going to Miss Molly's class when you were three? You did ballet and you got to wear that pretty tutu."

"I don't want to."

"Well, how about basketball? Do you want to try that?"

"No."

"How about swimming?"

"No."

I can't explain why I just let her say no. I wish I could go back in time and stop asking for her permission. I was the parent; she was a five-year-old. She didn't know how to make good choices, so it was up to me to step up and make those decisions on her behalf. But I didn't. I just wanted her to be happy.

• • •

Dan and I didn't want Breanna to feel bad about herself, so we didn't talk to her about her weight. We knew that other kids would make her fully aware of her size soon enough. At every opportunity, I told her, "God made you special. You're so beautiful and kind. You're always going to be our precious daughter."

The nutritionist came by the house a few times. I implemented some of his suggestions, such as taking away a few of the fattier foods and including more fruits and vegetables into Breanna's meals. He also told me to quit cooking with cream of mushroom soup. I did, but food seemed flavorless without it. He also advised us to eat several smaller meals rather than three big meals each day. This plan went over like a bag of rocks.

"I'm hungry, Mommy!" Brenna said at the end of a meal.

"No more for now."

"But . . . but . . ."

Oh, the tears! She would cry and cry, telling me how empty her tummy felt. Even though I knew she had just eaten, I still felt bad for her. *She's a big girl*, I rationalized. *She needs more food than most people to fill up.* How do you say no when your child is hungry? It just didn't seem right.

Even so, I continued with the nutritionist's basic plan. A few weeks later he came back and measured her body fat again using skin-fold calipers.

"This is good," he said. "Her body fat percentage is going down."

Really? She looked exactly the same to me. It didn't seem like much of a reward for all those tears.

The nutritionist hadn't given us a specific written plan, just a bunch of tips. These strategies would have been common sense for most people, but they were utterly foreign to me. Did people really fill half their plates with fruits and vegetables? How could chicken taste good if it wasn't breaded and fried? I attempted healthy cooking a couple of times, but Breanna totally rejected it, and truth be told, I didn't like it either. I also bought sprouted wheat bread instead of white bread, based on the nutritionist's suggestion. We all had the same reaction: *Gross!* It was such a different taste and texture from what we were used to.

Nobody could like this stuff, I told myself. *Why would someone put seeds in bread?*

We wanted to eat like normal people. I was convinced that all normal people with kids cooked the way I did and served their thin kids the same foods I did.

Slowly but surely, the old habits crept right back in. The nutritionist's advice went by the wayside, and the corn dogs and creamy pastas took their place at the lunch table once more. Now I know what a big mistake I was making, but at the time I was focused on the short term. When Breanna was eating, she was happy (and so were we). I was pretty sure I would never buy sprouted wheat bread again as long as we lived. *Good riddance. Welcome home, white bread and dinner rolls.*

• • •

Breanna didn't make eye contact when she ate. She guarded her food as if someone might steal it at any moment, and she devoured everything at startling speeds. I wasn't sure she was even enjoying the food as much as inhaling it.

I didn't realize how different she was from other kids until I was babysitting a few friends' kids and noticed the way they picked at their food. They were eating mostly the same things Breanna ate, but in a completely different way. Two bites of this, three bites of that, and then they wanted to run off and play again. Breanna

What if Your Child Refuses to Eat New (Healthy) Foods?

Research shows that you may need to try a new food up to ten times before you can really decide if you like it or not. So if at first you or your children hate every vegetable on the plate, that's a normal reaction. You have to commit to serving each new food ten times before making an accurate judgment.

Here's a deal you can make with your children: they have to try a new food ten times before they can say they don't like it. But keep in mind it has to be ten *different* times, not ten bites at the same meal. If they still don't like it after they've tried it ten times, then they don't have to try it again for another few months.

You can keep a chart to show how many times they've tried each food. And it works for grown-ups, too!

would clean her plate and then want more—and she didn't really care about running off to play. She preferred activities that could be done while sitting or standing in one place: artwork, singing, playing with dolls.

When one of the girls saw the way Breanna ate, she said, "Gosh, Breanna, calm down. No one's going to take it away from you."

Not only was she focused on her meals while she was eating them, but she also seemed to be consumed by thoughts of food outside of mealtimes. Soon after breakfast, she wanted to know what we were having for lunch. Right after lunch, she was thinking about dinner. And on days when she had friends over, she knew there was a possibility we'd make cupcakes.

I liked entertaining and having friends over, and we would always put out plenty of fattening foods and desserts. It was essentially a giant buffet of fried, stuffed, breaded, sautéed, and otherwise calorie-laden foods. The grown-ups would spend time talking to one another while the kids played. I rarely supervised what Breanna ate on those days.

"Breanna just filled up a whole plate with rice pilaf," one of my friends warned me at a get-together.

I sighed. *What am I supposed to do?* I wondered. I couldn't fathom going back to the rules the nutritionist had imposed— it had been way too stressful listening to my daughter whine and cry all day long. But what was the alternative? I knew that if this pattern continued, my child was heading toward a life of obesity. We had to find a way to break the cycle.

"What should we do?" I asked Dan that night.

"I don't know," he said. "I just don't know."

• • •

That's where we kept getting stuck: somewhere between "There's a problem" and "What do we do about it?" We'd make changes, but we were inconsistent in enforcing them. One day I'd put my foot down and tell Breanna to put away the bag of chips, and the next day I'd let her help herself to another serving. I didn't want to be a mean mom. And I hated to see my child feeling deprived or sad.

When we had family dinners, Dan's mother would serve up the most delectable baked goods—an assortment of pastries that even a supermodel couldn't resist. Of course I didn't want to tell my mother-in-law to stop baking for us. And again, I didn't believe this was the problem. Surely an occasional splurge on dessert wasn't at fault for my daughter's weight, so I didn't make it a priority to put an end to it.

As Breanna's year of kindergarten wore on, I thought often about what would happen with her peers as she got older. Would she be teased in school because of her weight? It hadn't happened yet that year, but I knew that kids became crueler as they got older. I also worried that she would be at risk for type 2 diabetes, which was the only health risk I associated with obesity. Dan's father had had diabetes and had died young as a result of complications from the disease.

One day I expressed my concerns to a friend.

"You should see this holistic doctor I know," my friend said. "She has an overweight daughter too, so she'll understand."

Her words gave me hope. I called to schedule an appointment, but the holistic doctor was booked for six months. It was a long time to wait, and during those months, I built up this doctor in my mind—I was sure she would give us the answer we'd been looking for. Per Breanna's request, her dad took her to the appointment, and I stayed home with Nathan.

Finally, after all the waiting and all the buildup . . . the doctor had nothing. I guess I should have thought more about the fact that her daughter was overweight too: it wasn't that she'd been overweight in the past and had gotten over it, but she was currently overweight. If the doctor couldn't help her own daughter, I'm not sure why I thought she could help us.

The doctor's only suggestion was that we take Breanna to a psychologist. That didn't feel right to me. Breanna had been overeating since she was a baby; surely there weren't deep-rooted issues that would cause her to overeat at just one year old.

It was another defeat. Dan walked out of the office feeling like we'd wasted a lot of time—not to mention hope.

"God, please point us in the right direction," I prayed. "We need an answer. I know this isn't good for Breanna. Help us find the right doctor who will know what to do."

I thought the answer would have to come from medical professionals. After all, they were the experts on health, with degrees from esteemed schools to prove it. Who was I? Just a mom. I had not yet accepted that for Breanna, as for most people, the answer was simple, if not easy: it was all about diet and exercise. But at the time, I was convinced we just hadn't knocked on the right professional's door yet. And so I went off to knock on some more.

. . .

Maybe it's a food allergy, I thought. *If she's reacting to a particular type of food, it may be causing her to gain weight.* I was grasping at straws, but I wasn't sure what else to do.

We made an appointment with an allergist, but once we got there we found out that the doctor was only qualified to do skin testing for environmental allergies. We discovered that she was allergic to grass and olive trees, but that didn't help us with her weight.

My dad knew a specialist in Emeryville who could do the food allergy testing, so we made the three-hour drive to have blood tests done. This was an adult practice, though, and they didn't have much experience dealing with children. After lots of poking and prodding, they eventually said, "We're sorry, but we just can't find a vein."

Dan asked them to fax over paperwork to our local children's hospital so her blood could be drawn there. Breanna hated needles, so we bribed her into going by telling her she could have breakfast at IHOP with Daddy the morning of the testing. Once again, we hit a dead end when the report came back showing that she had no allergies that would explain her weight gain.

At the time, my concerns about Breanna's weight centered on the social implications she'd face, with a side helping of worry over the possibility of diabetes. What I didn't know was that there are countless problems related to childhood obesity that she was already experiencing or could experience in the near future. Being overweight or obese affects a child's development in every way—physical, emotional, and spiritual—and it can have long-lasting effects.

What's more, the earlier someone becomes obese, the earlier these problems kick in. In other words, someone who becomes obese as an adult will likely have more time before they experience serious health effects, whereas kids' bodies are more vulnerable. Since they are still maturing, obesity

Medical Conditions Associated with Obesity
- high blood pressure (which can lead to heart disease)
- high cholesterol (which can lead to heart disease)
- asthma
- early-onset arthritis (due to excessive weight on joints, which wears away cartilage)
- broken bones
- damage to growth plates, leading to malformed bones
- severely bowed legs (Blount's disease)
- gallstones
- gastroesophageal reflux
- snoring (which leads to poor sleep)
- sleep apnea (leads to poor sleep as well as daytime effects similar to those from long-term sleep deprivation)
- flat feet (which can cause walking to be painful)
- surgical complications (longer healing times, side effects from anesthesia, and greater risk for additional invasive medical intervention)
- slipped capital femoral epiphysis (which occurs when the hip bone disconnects from the thigh bone and the thigh bone slips backward)
- stunted growth
- fatty liver disease
- metabolic syndrome (which increases the risk of heart disease, stroke, and diabetes)
- increased risk of cancer
- fatigue
- early onset of puberty
- low self-esteem
- depression

can permanently interfere with normal development. Extra weight on bones and joints means that they may never grow as they should.

I am convinced that if I'd known these things, I would have taken Breanna's weight more seriously. As it was, it was something I took seriously *sometimes*. I took it seriously enough to talk to my friends and family about it, take her to doctors, hide junk food on occasion, and make periodic attempts to get her into sports.

Our latest halfhearted attempts on the sports front were T-ball (which didn't require much exercise at all) and a children's fitness class at a franchise gym, which turned out to be more about playing and getting an introduction to gym equipment than about actual fitness. It wasn't geared toward weight loss; it was pretty much a babysitting service for parents who wanted to work out at the gym.

When we went to Disneyland as a family, we'd watch other kids running ahead of their parents, unable to wait for the next ride. Breanna, on the other hand, lagged behind us. When I took her for a pony ride, she had to go on a full-sized horse. It was heartbreaking to see this little girl on a horse for grown-ups, not knowing why she was different from the other kids her age.

In spite of the weight-related worries in the background, Breanna remained a happy kid overall. She couldn't keep up with the other kids, but it didn't seem to bother her. I regularly checked for signs that she was being teased or that she was unhappy, but they weren't there. She didn't see herself as a "fat kid"—just a kid. And thankfully, she had a few friends and one best friend who sometimes came over to spend the night.

Maybe I'm worrying for nothing, I thought. I knew that having friends could help shield her from the pain of bullying, so I did what I could to make sure she had plenty of opportunities to meet other kids and form friendships. Our house was always stocked with chocolate milk, ingredients for baking, and extra boxes of macaroni and cheese just in case we had the opportunity for playdates.

I hoped it would always be that way.

EAT THIS INSTEAD OF THAT

Making healthy food choices doesn't have to feel overwhelming, and it doesn't necessarily mean scrapping everything you and your family are used to eating. Sometimes it's just a matter of making smart choices and replacing foods with their healthier counterparts, one at a time.

What to Avoid	What to Eat Instead
potato chips/corn chips	kale chips, collard greens chips, carrot/celery sticks, rice cakes, homemade chips
regular meatballs	ground turkey meatballs or extra-lean beef meatballs
butter/margarine	broth (for cooking); powdered peanut butter (for toast)
regular yogurt (whether it's fat free or not)	fat-free Greek yogurt
sugar	no-sugar-added applesauce, honey
mashed potatoes	mashed cauliflower
white bread	sprouted whole-grain bread
chicken nuggets	grilled chicken strips
whole milk	nonfat milk
cream cheese	low-fat cottage cheese or Greek yogurt
canned cream-based soups	broth-based soups

What to Avoid	What to Eat Instead
white rice	brown rice
microwave popcorn	air-popped popcorn
white hamburger buns	whole-wheat pitas
candy	sunflower seeds or a serving of raisins
mayonnaise	hummus
juice/soda	water/tea

CHAPTER 3

CHILDHOOD LOST

BETWEEN THE AGES OF THREE AND NINE, we shuttled Breanna from one doctor to another who ran one set of tests after another. Sometimes we went to multiple doctors in one month; other times months elapsed in between. But even if we weren't actively doing something to address it, her weight was always hovering in a corner of my mind. As she got older, she just kept getting bigger, and in a worrying turn of events, so did her little brother. By the time he was two, it looked as if he might follow in her footsteps.

When Breanna was at Valley Children's Hospital getting tested for food allergies, the nurse who was drawing blood asked Dan why they were there. When Dan explained about Breanna's appetite, he said, "That sounds like an endocrinology problem, not an allergy."

I was happy to have another avenue to try. We called the endocrinology department the next day and scheduled an appointment. Dan took Breanna to her appointment to check for genetic disorders such as Prader-Willi syndrome—a rare condition that causes poor muscle tone and an insatiable appetite in children.

I'd seen an episode of *Oprah* about the syndrome but didn't think this could be what Breanna was dealing with since the symptoms also include behavior problems, short stature, and cognitive disabilities—none of which described Breanna. When the results came back, and she was again given a clean bill of health, I felt a strange mix of relief and disappointment. I was thankful she didn't have a genetic disorder, but it was difficult to not get any answers.

"She doesn't have diabetes . . . yet," the doctor said, "But she will. I just had to break that news to the parents of my last patient. Based on Breanna's charts, it looks like she's gaining twenty pounds each year. If she keeps going like this, diabetes will be inevitable."

When Dan got home, he told me what the doctor had said.

"But she doesn't have diabetes yet, right?"

That was a glimmer of good news, but we still had no answers for the future.

The doctor must think I'm a bad mother, I thought. *I'm sure he assumes I don't care. But I do. I'm going to keep searching until we find an answer.*

It frustrated me that so much time was passing with no improvement to Breanna's weight—and no real plan to fix the problem. But there was something else that was troubling me: my little girl was changing in more ways than just her body shape.

. . .

The last time I'd seen Breanna as a happy, normal kid was at about age five or six. After that, things started to get darker. She withdrew from people. She was no longer excited to see her friends and go to school. She didn't want to do anything that involved movement. We kept signing her up for activities in the hope that she'd find something she enjoyed—our two latest attempts were baseball and tumbling, and we took her to Pump It Up to play on the inflatable bouncers. We had no success—the only sport that interested her was cheerleading. She'd been involved in a workshop for a cheerleading camp in kindergarten and loved it, but by second grade, that no longer seemed like a possibility for her. She just couldn't move like the other girls. I couldn't imagine what it would be like for her as a teenager to try to squeeze into a cheerleading uniform and join in their acrobatic routines, flipping and leaping in the air. Breanna was *not* a leaper. She was more of a stand-stiller.

In almost all respects, both my kids were easy to parent. Nathan was a happy toddler and a good sleeper, and Breanna was an obedient student who never caused her teachers trouble. Nathan looked up to his big sister and copied everything she did, which was a good thing . . . except when it came to her junk food habits.

Breanna never mentioned her weight. She wasn't down on herself—and to be honest, she didn't even appear to notice. It seemed that when Breanna looked in a mirror, she saw a girl of normal weight. Sometimes I wondered if that was because I'd drilled into her mind that God had made her perfect just the way she was. Was it possible that my pep talks had gone too far and now she would think that an obese body was perfect?

There was only one time I remember Breanna even hinting at discomfort with her body. When she was in the bathtub one day, she said, "It hurts! It really hurts right here." She pointed at her stomach. "There's a lot of pressure." I looked at where she was pointing and saw the part of her stomach that was all stretched out and supporting the excess weight. Did she understand that this wasn't normal? That most kids didn't hurt because of extra layers of fat?

I cried that night, feeling more helpless than ever. Like so many other nights, I looked ahead to Breanna's future, and it wasn't a pretty sight. If she was hurting now, what would her life be like in twenty years, when she was an adult? If she hated to move now, would she ever get up off the couch once she had the choice not to? Was my beautiful girl going to wind up a reclusive homebody who never went anywhere? It was a devastating thought, and I pushed it out of my mind as fast as I could.

But I had to admit to myself that she wasn't the same person she used to be. The little girl who used to dance and sing all over the living room—who used to be filled with laughter and carefree silliness—was slipping away. I felt like I was watching the light in her eyes go dim.

"Is anyone bothering you at school?" I asked. "You know you can tell us anything."

"No, I'm fine," she'd say.

It was impossible to get much more than that out of her. Every time we asked, she'd reassure us that no one was bothering her. It was hard for me to believe, but I wasn't sure how else to find out what was going on.

I knew how Dan had been teased as a child, and I knew that our society hadn't gotten better since we were kids. Every time I heard stories of inventive ways kids were finding to bully each other—such as through the Internet and cell phones—in addition to the old standbys of physical bullying, name calling, verbal abuse, and social exclusion, I shuddered to think that Breanna could be a target.

The truth is that kids will find any reason to pick on one another, whether they decide someone is too tall, too short, too quiet, or too awkward. When I was a kid, it was something as silly as my last name: Dorfmeier. It got turned into a dozen stupid nicknames that followed me all through school—Dorkmeier, Dorfus, Oscar Meyer. As trivial as that was, it chipped away at my self-esteem. I felt like an outcast at school. I fell in with a rougher group of kids who liked to ditch class, and I eventually wound up at a special continuation high school for troubled kids. It took me until adulthood to repair the damage and realize that what other people said or thought about me didn't in any way define who I really was. What mattered was the content of my character.

I also knew that being overweight is one of the easiest ways for kids to get picked on, because it's something they can't hide. And while there have been big movements to get people to understand that racism and sexism are wrong, fat-shaming is still alive and well. It's one of the few areas of bullying that's still socially acceptable, even among adults.

Adults who would never use derogatory words against some-one's race or gender might look at someone at the beach and comment under their breath, "What a whale" or "I can't believe she's wearing that."

Overweight adults may be overlooked for job promotions and leadership positions, and they are often thought of as lazy. Alcoholics can sleep off their drunkenness; heroin addicts can hide their track marks. People who are addicted to food, how-ever, can't cover up their struggle for any part of the day. But at least adults have some say in what kind of job they do, and who they'll choose to be around on a daily basis. Kids don't get that choice. They're stuck in a classroom with the same kids each day, and if any of those kids happens to be mean—and odds are pretty good that there will be at least one bully in each class—then guess who makes an easy target?

More than half of all overweight or obese high school students in the United States say that they're bullied about their weight on a daily basis.[1] In many cases that can lead to depression and even suicidal thoughts.

As I watched my daughter's weight climb, I became more aware of those kinds of stories in the news. Ashlynn Connor, a ten-year-old in Illinois, hanged herself by a scarf in her closet because her classmates had called her "fat" and "ugly."[2] Two fourteen-year-old best friends died in a suicide pact in Minnesota in 2011 after months of being bullied about their weight and appearance.[3]

The thought of something like that happening to Breanna one day nearly paralyzed me.

From what I had observed, she wasn't being bullied yet, but I was always on the alert. *Something* was causing a change in her personality. Fewer and fewer girls came by our house to play with Breanna anymore; by the time she was in second grade, there was only one friend Breanna talked about. She didn't speak badly about the other kids; she just didn't seem to connect with any of them. I watched the other kids talking and giggling together after school, and I knew right away that my daughter was an outsider. Birthday invitations that once came frequently when everyone in the class was invited were now few and far between. Sometimes Breanna would hear about these parties while she was at school, and she'd come home and tell me about it.

"Everyone was talking about going to Janie's party this Saturday," she said. "But I didn't get invited."

"I'm sorry, honey," I told her. "Janie doesn't know what she's missing."

I wasn't sure which one of us was hurt more by this ostracism. As a parent, I desperately wanted my daughter to belong—to feel happy and secure.

Can't the other kids see her? I cried out silently. *There's so much more to her than her size.*

It seemed that Breanna was losing her ability to interact with her peers. She was so quiet—not only with us, but in school, too. The shield she'd had around her in the form of playmates was disappearing. Now we were her only shield, and we couldn't be there all the time. I felt helpless to do anything except pray.

"Maybe she'll open up more to you," I said to Dan. "You know what it was like to be a kid with weight struggles."

"I'll talk to her," he agreed.

She had no problem opening up to him about her physical

complaints—like the fact that she was developing rashes under her belly rolls and that her thighs were chafing. But she still didn't talk about any problems with kids at school.

Dan suggested that I put baby powder under her rolls to soak up perspiration and keep her dry. The powder gave her some relief, but she still had rashes, so the doctor prescribed a cream. When I pointed out the stretch marks all over her body, he prescribed another cream for that. But as willing as he was to write out prescription after prescription for weight-related problems, he remained unwilling to talk about weight loss.

"If you want to do something for her," he said, "wait until she's sixteen and then put her on a crash diet. If you have her diet before then, you'll stunt her growth."

That sounded ridiculous to me. How could it be safe to gain weight and unsafe to lose it?

When Breanna was seven, I'd learned about a summer camp for kids who wanted to lose weight, but at $7,000 for two weeks, it was well beyond our budget. I called anyway, trying to plead my case.

"Do you have any scholarships or financial aid?" I asked. "My daughter really needs help, and I don't know what else to do."

The receptionist was nice, but she couldn't reduce the price. I called again the next year, hoping they'd change their mind. They didn't.

Now another year had passed, and we were worse off than ever. Dan and I talked about the camp idea again. Could we save up enough to send Breanna? I'd read so many success stories on their website by parents who said this camp had solved their weight problems. It was tempting, but it sounded too good to be true. How could two weeks make that much of a difference? Was that long enough to make real lifestyle changes?

We decided to sign her up for a summer sports camp instead. Unfortunately, she hurt her foot early on and never went back. We made yet another trek to the doctor, who told us to get orthopedic inserts for her shoes. Apparently her arches were failing and making her feet flat. He didn't

Reading Labels: Beware of the Fine Print

If something says it's "low fat," you first have to ask yourself, *Compared to what?* Let's say a candy bar has eighteen grams of fat, and of that, eleven grams are saturated fat. If that candy company figures out a way to cut down the fat to thirteen grams, including eleven grams of saturated fat, that company can now call this candy bar "reduced fat" since it has almost 30 percent less fat than the regular version. But guess what? That's still a ridiculous amount of fat for a snack!

Where it gets even uglier is when you find out what happened to make those extra five grams of fat disappear. The fat wasn't just cut out, with everything else still in place. Nope. Fat is in processed foods because it makes them taste good— or at least, that's what we're used to as "good." In place of the fat, other chemicals are added to give the product more flavor—and you won't know that unless you pay attention to the ingredients list.

Here are some of the sweeteners to avoid: aspartame, sucralose, and xylitol. All have potentially dangerous side effects, ranging from digestive problems to migraines to an inability to regulate blood sugar. And artificial sweeteners, even when they result in lower amounts of calories, don't solve the underlying problem of an addiction to sugary sweetness. Break the cycle, and your kids will develop a taste for real foods that aren't loaded with sugar and chemicals.

say what was causing the problem, but now the answer is obvious: it was all the extra weight she was carrying around.

. . .

One of Breanna's favorite things to do was to cook with me. Ever since she was a toddler, she'd loved helping in the kitchen, climbing up on a chair to help me stir mashed potatoes. I remember how proud she was when she learned how to crack eggs without my help.

I could still count on her help as I made pancakes for breakfast on the weekends. Pancakes were a particular favorite, and she'd regularly devour an entire stack. I reasoned that she needed a big breakfast (it was the most important meal of the day, after all) so she'd be able to keep her energy up throughout the day. But I decided it was time to take small steps to improve the ingredients in Breanna's meals. I kept cooking as usual for the rest of the family, but for her portions, I combed the grocery store for products labeled "low fat," "fat free," "nonfat," "diet," "light," and "low calorie."

Reading Labels: Serving Sizes

It's important to pay attention not only to the fat, sugar, and calories on a food label but also to the size of the servings. It won't do you a lot of good to pick out something low in fat and then serve your child twice as much.

Serving sizes, it should be noted, are *not recommended* serving sizes. They're supposed to represent the average amount that people will eat in one sitting. Unfortunately, food labels don't always offer an accurate reflection. For instance, half a cup is the serving size for ice cream. Who do you know who eats half a cup of ice cream? Or one chocolate chip cookie? Or fifteen chips?

I fell for the hype. If the package said anything about it being helpful for weight loss, I believed it. I'm sure marketing teams loved people like me. I assumed those labels guaranteed that the product was healthier than the regular version and would actually help Breanna lose weight.

What I didn't know at the time is that most of those claims mean nothing. If anything, they mark the things you should probably *avoid*. The thing is, there's a lot of spin when it comes to food packaging. The hype you read on the front of the package often doesn't match what you'll find out if you really pay attention to the nutrition labels—and I didn't. It wasn't that I didn't care, but I hadn't yet learned what those labels actually meant, so even if I had read them, I would have had no idea what I was reading.

Back then, I didn't realize that "low fat" often means "we added a ton of sugar and other chemicals because it didn't taste any good without the fat." I didn't know that some foods labeled "fat free" have even more calories than their full-fat counterparts, or that some of the products marketed as diet foods are based on such small serving sizes that no one actually eats just one serving—which means their "diet" goes right out the window!

I had no idea that I should pay attention not only to the amount of sugar in a product but also to artificial sweeteners, which may be even more harmful than sugar. A recent study showed that the use of artificial sweeteners led to excessive bacteria in the digestive system and glucose intolerance.[4]

And I thought that chicken nuggets were actually, you know, *chicken*. I never would have guessed that only one out of the twenty-five ingredients in some chicken nuggets is actually chicken. I thought chicken sounded healthier than cheeseburgers, so I figured that was a pretty good choice for the kids when we went out to eat. I really didn't even know what people meant when they talked about "processed" food. When I was growing up, food was food. We didn't analyze it—we just ate it!

It was foreign territory for me to buy products that sounded like diet foods, but it seemed like the right next step. So instead of giving Breanna fried tortilla chips, I gave her baked chips—a much better option, I was convinced. In fact, since they were so much healthier, I didn't worry about her having seconds or thirds.

And yet the numbers on the scale kept climbing. It was maddening.

We didn't have her weigh in with much regularity—we just did it every few months when we thought about it. I'd never seen the number go down or even stay the same for Breanna—or Nathan either, for that matter. Breanna was the bigger problem, but I knew that Nathan was following in her steps. Already he was transitioning from a chubby toddler to a seriously overweight preschooler.

"Why is this happening?" I cried out to Dan one night. "I'm buying her all the right food!"

"I don't know," Dan said. "I guess it's just not enough. We have to monitor her more."

If only he'd known how prophetic those words were.

• • •

When Breanna was in second grade, I got a notice in her backpack informing me that her cafeteria funds were depleted, and I'd have to send in more money. Now I'll admit that keeping track of money is not one of my strongest points. I handle bills as they come in, but I'm not always as watchful as I should be. This time, though, I was sure it was too soon to pay again, so I called the school.

"I just got a note saying that Breanna needs more money in her lunch account," I said. "But that doesn't seem right. Didn't I just pay $50 a couple of weeks ago?"

"Yes, ma'am, you did."

"Then how is it all gone? The price of school lunch didn't go up, did it?"

"No, it's still the same. And breakfast, too."

"Well, she doesn't eat breakfast at school. She eats at home."

There was a long pause.

"Are you sure about that, Mrs. Bond?"

"What do you mean?"

"The records I have here show that she eats breakfast at school every day."

"No, that's wrong. She eats here. It's just lunch that she . . ."

Now it was my turn to pause. What was this woman telling me?

"Wait, are you saying that she's been eating breakfast when she gets to school? How is that possible?"

"When she comes in, she picks up breakfast in the cafeteria before class. The bus gets in early for the kids who eat before class."

My mind was swirling, and I could barely get any words out. "Thank you," I finally choked out. "I'll need to talk to Breanna about this."

The day couldn't pass quickly enough. Suddenly everything made sense! No wonder those numbers on the scale were still climbing.

When Breanna got home from school, I said, "Hey,

honey, can I ask you something? When you get to school in the morning, are you going to the cafeteria and getting breakfast?"

She looked at her shoes and nodded.

"Well, you can't do that anymore. You eat breakfast at home with us every day. You're not supposed to eat another breakfast at school. Do you understand?"

She looked so sad, as if I'd taken away her favorite doll. It hurt me to see such a forlorn look on her face.

A few weeks later, I talked to a family friend whose son was in Breanna's class. Her son had told her that Breanna was asking other kids for food at lunch. Some of her classmates had prepackaged snacks that they hadn't eaten—Goldfish crackers, cookies, chips—and she would collect any extras they didn't want. I was heartbroken to hear this latest development. Why was my child so desperate for food all the time?

When I told Breanna that this pattern, too, needed to stop, she didn't cry or make a big deal about it like she would have a couple of years before. Instead, she didn't say a word. When I saw the look of defeat on her face, I found myself wishing for the old Breanna, whining and all.

• • •

"Dan, this is why she's still gaining weight!" I was relieved to finally have an answer. "She's been eating two breakfasts and extra snacks every day at school!"

"It's a good thing we found out," he agreed.

We both assumed that after a month or two, we'd start to see the numbers on the scale go down. But it didn't happen. Her weight kept climbing, just as quickly as it had before. I was aggravated—why wasn't anything working? How was it possible that nothing we were doing was making a difference?

On some level, I knew that I had to get Breanna moving more, but exercise was just so hard for her. She moved slowly and uncomfortably, with labored breaths. And then there was the matter of what she could even wear if she did something active.

We'd long ago given up on shopping in the children's department at clothing stores, and we were down to very few options. JCPenney had a plus-size department for kids, but she outgrew it by age eight. Stores like Wet Seal, Macy's, and Justice weren't even worth walking into anymore.

By chance, we discovered that she could fit into the extra-extra-large T-shirts we found at a craft store, so we bought one in every color. Her only choices to go with the T-shirts were skirts or sweatpants with elastic waistbands. I tried to compensate for her limited wardrobe by making sure she had her hair done nicely, with bows and ribbons and braids, but she still couldn't participate in the latest fashions like the other girls in school could. They were all shopping at Justice, and she was shopping at Michael's.

When I had my baby girl, I had visions in my head of all the adorable outfits I would buy for her. I certainly never imagined a wardrobe that consisted entirely of big T-shirts and elastic-waistband pants.

Even though we'd managed to find clothes that fit, Breanna wasn't truly comfortable. She was a child living in the body of an obese adult, and she was having more and more trouble completing the simplest physical tasks. How would things ever change?

I felt inadequate as a mother for not being able to figure this out for her and get it under control.

Worst of all, my sweet girl was losing her spark. I didn't know if it had anything to do with her weight or not—she didn't complain about her appearance—but I felt her vibrant personality gradually disappearing. It was like seeing her shadow—a more withdrawn, less enthusiastic version of the person she used to be. All those times she'd sung and danced in the middle of the living room, all the times I'd watched her make friends on the playground . . . Where had those moments gone?

And more important, how could I get my daughter back?

CHECKLIST TO IDENTIFY DEPRESSION

There is a strong link between childhood obesity and depression, and the longer a child is overweight, the higher his or her risk for depression. It can be difficult for parents to know whether their child is just going through a moody stage or is actually depressed. The American Academy of Child and Adolescent Psychiatry offers these warning signs:[5]

- ❑ Does your child experience frequent bouts of crying?
- ❑ Does your child show a decreased interest in favorite activities?
- ❑ Does your child express feelings of hopelessness?
- ❑ Is your child persistently bored, with low energy?
- ❑ Is your child isolated from peers?
- ❑ Does your child have poor communication skills when interacting with peers?
- ❑ Does your child make statements that reflect low self-esteem and guilt?

- ❑ Is your child extremely sensitive to rejection or failure?
- ❑ Is your child more irritable, angry, or hostile than usual?
- ❑ Is your child struggling in most relationships?
- ❑ Does your child frequently complain of physical illnesses such as headaches and stomachaches?
- ❑ Does your child frequently ask to stay home from school?
- ❑ Has your child's performance in school declined?
- ❑ Does your child have difficulty concentrating?
- ❑ Have you noticed a major change in your child's eating and/or sleeping patterns?
- ❑ Does your child talk about trying to run away from home?
- ❑ Does your child express suicidal thoughts?
- ❑ Does your child exhibit self-destructive behavior?

It's important not to ignore signs of depression or to assume your child will eventually get over it. Don't be afraid to ask straight out: "Are you sad? Are you having a hard time? Can you think of anything that might make it better?"

Also, if you suspect that your child needs more help than you can provide, don't hesitate to seek help. You may want to ask your doctor, school counselor, or pastor for recommendations of child or family psychologists or counselors who can help.

CHAPTER 4

SUGAR FIX

BREANNA HAD ALWAYS WANTED to take the bus to school. When she was three years old, every time a school bus passed our house, she'd say, "Mommy, I want to ride the bus!"

At the time I'd told her that she was too young, and she'd get to ride the bus when she got older. But now that she was in her early primary school years, I started to feel protective. I didn't like the idea of her being largely unsupervised with a bunch of kids, most of whom were older than she was. If I noticed that Breanna was different from other girls her age, then surely her peers noticed. I was afraid she'd be an easy target.

I would have been fine picking her up and dropping her off all the way through high school, but she still wanted the experience of riding the bus. So when she was in third grade, I finally—reluctantly—agreed. She wasn't making friends readily in school, so I thought maybe the bus would be a way to meet other kids.

After seeing her off at the bus stop, I'd go home and get on the computer. Almost every day, I'd spend the morning researching childhood obesity. I was desperate for a plan—a formula I could follow. I searched for personal stories and before-and-after photos that would inspire us, but there wasn't much out there. There were plenty of websites dedicated to adults who wanted to lose weight, but the information pertaining to kids was limited.

And most of what I did find was depressing. I read the studies about how obese kids were more likely to have psychological problems—from suicidal thoughts to poor self-esteem—as well as a wide range of physical problems, many of which Breanna had already started experiencing. I started to question whether she had ever needed that tonsillectomy or whether her sleeping problems had been strictly weight related.

My research also made me worry about what else lay ahead. So far it had been just about a miracle that her health was as good as it was, considering her difficulty breathing and moving. She even managed to have perfect attendance at school—although that may have been a sad commentary on how little she interacted with other kids. She didn't pick up their germs, but she also didn't get close enough to them to have meaningful friendships.

. . .

Just when I was starting to feel utterly alone in our journey, I found a wonderful group of friends through Nathan's kindergarten. The parents of his classmates would hang around and talk at pickup and drop-off times, and we became a tight-knit group.

I babysat the son of one of my friends, and over time his mom and I became close. One evening when she came to pick him up, I confided in her about my struggles with Breanna's weight.

"I bet my daughter would love to work out with her," she said.

That sounded like a fantastic idea. Her daughter was a junior in high school, and I hired her two or three days a week to exercise with Breanna. The plan was for them to go on bike rides and do other kid-friendly workouts. I was hoping this would finally be the answer we needed for her to lose weight.

I should have known that it was doomed from the start.

They'd bike for just a couple of blocks, and then Breanna would simply stop.

"She wouldn't move," the girl told me. "She just quit in the middle of the road and refused to go anywhere."

"Listen, Breanna, you have to give it a shot," I said.

The girl kept trying, but the result was the same every time: within minutes, Breanna would give a list of reasons why she couldn't go any farther—often accompanied by tears.

It was hot.

Her legs hurt.

She was tired.

It was too hard.

After a few sessions, Breanna told me that she didn't want to go anymore.

"You have to go," I said.

The older girl made a valiant effort. Each day she'd muster

up as much motivation as she could and try to get Breanna to go a reasonable distance. But there was no progress from day to day or week to week. Finally, as Breanna sat crying on the side of the road beside her bike one day, a car pulled over.

"Are you okay?" the driver asked. "It looks like you might need medical attention."

That marked the end of the bike rides. It was hard on my friend's daughter—and pointless for us.

I didn't know where to turn next. I cried out to God, "Do something here. I'm failing. I need you to step in and help us."

I hadn't recognized yet that *I* was the one causing the problem. The fatty comfort foods, the lack of limits, the cabinets stocked with junk food, the months of television and no physical activity—all of those patterns were having disastrous effects. I thought we could turn it around by making a few little changes, but it was too late for that. Breanna was in the third grade, and she already weighed more than 160 pounds.

"You know that God made you beautiful, right?" I would ask her regularly. "You're such a pretty girl."

I wanted my voice to be the one she would carry with her when others were not as kind with their words. I'd seen the looks and the whispers she got now when we went out in public. Other people didn't see her the way I did; all they saw was fat.

It was a word Breanna abhorred, though she rarely talked about it. We were at the dinner table one day when Nathan used the word *fat* in conversation. I don't remember what we were talking about, but I do know we never used the word *fat* in a derogatory way.

"Mom! He used the word *fat*!" Breanna exploded. Then she turned to him. "Don't ever say that word! I never want to hear that word ever again!"

We all went silent. Since that time on the playground back when she was a toddler, she'd never shown any signs that she even recognized she was overweight or that this word could be hurtful to her. Her words hung in the air—a warning to all of us that there was more going on than we could see.

What I didn't know at the time was that Breanna was being made fun of at school—she was being called "fathead" and "ugly" on the playground and other times when teachers weren't in close proximity. At the end of the year, Breanna's school had a talent show, and she sang with a couple of her friends. Before she started, someone said, "She's going to break the stage!" and the laughter spread like wildfire. Soon all the kids were looking at her and giggling.

For Breanna, that type of comment was nothing new, except that this time it felt like the whole school was in on it. It felt like everyone was laughing at her, not just the individual bullies who had called her names. I wouldn't hear about the talent show incident until about six months afterward, when one of her friends mentioned it casually in front of me.

It was shaping up to be a long year.

• • •

Even the simple routine of getting ready in the morning was a struggle. Seeing Breanna in the bathtub was a daily wake-up call. We had a recessed tub, and she struggled to get in and out. I'd sit with her and wash her hair, and when she was finished, she'd have to grab my arm to balance and navigate her legs over the side of the tub. As I watched her struggle with her limited range of motion, it was like watching what an elderly person would go through.

Both Dan and I were becoming exhausted from the battle. Every time we thought we were moving in the right direction, there were more temptations and setbacks. "Kid culture," as it turned out, was a force to be reckoned with. I had never before considered how much our culture encourages giving junk food to kids. Halloween, of course, is the most indulgent holiday when it comes to candy and sweets, but it seemed that nearly every day there was some kind of celebration or excuse to give out junk food. At school, there were all the class birthdays, accompanied by cookies and cupcakes as big as softballs, as well as coupons for free sundaes for doing well on a report card or completing a reading club. At home, there was the ice-cream truck jingling down the street and the neighbors selling Girl Scout cookies or candy bars for fund-raisers. Even store clerks handed out lollipops to well-behaved kids. Every day provided another opportunity for kids to eat garbage. It wasn't just offered, but encouraged. If I turned down candy for my children, people expected a reason. "You don't want a chocolate bar? Why not?"

I didn't have a consistent policy about these treats. Sometimes I refused on Breanna's behalf, but other times I didn't want her to feel like I was depriving her of a treat that all the other kids were allowed to have. She was always excited to bring home one of those coupons so we could go to a fast-food chain together to redeem her reward—and in the earlier years, I'd been happy to do it. But now I was starting to resent the barrage of unasked-for junk food.

"Mom, guess what we did in school today?"

"What?"

"We got to decorate our own cookies!"

"You did?"

I tried to sound excited, but the class had just had an ice-cream party the day before.

"Yes, and I made a flower and a sunshine on mine with icing! And then we got to put on the sprinkles! The cookies were so big!"

The problem wasn't limited to school, though—there was also the hairdresser who gave out candy for being good, the bank teller who gave kids butterscotch candies, and even the pediatrician who gave out gummy worms at the end of the visit.

Is it really any wonder that we're experiencing the largest obesity epidemic this country has ever seen? There is something very wrong when we're teaching our kids that junk food, which poisons their bodies, is a reward. "Rewards" are not supposed to give you diabetes and heart disease and sleep apnea. And these treats were undermining my efforts to cut down on my kids' junk food habits. People didn't ask if they could give my kids candy; they just did it. And if I tried to take it away, I was the bad guy.

I didn't want to be the bad guy.

It is startling to consider how much money corporations sink into marketing poisons to our kids. They research to figure out exactly how to package their junk: putting popular characters on the box, showing commercials during kids' favorite TV shows, putting it at their eye level at the checkout line, and making it look so appealing that they'll beg their parents to buy it right now! These companies do studies to figure out the exact amount of crunch a potato chip needs to make kids want to eat more, or how many marshmallows will get kids to crave more cereal. Food engineers conduct taste tests to find what the industry calls the "bliss point"—the just-right combination of ingredients so the consumer will not be satisfied quickly and will want more and more.[6]

As a result, we as a nation are eating more packaged junk than ever before—and in most cases, we don't even realize it's junk. For instance, most people think of yogurt as a healthy snack, and it was—once. But that was before companies started dumping extra sugar into their product and even adding chocolate and sprinkles and candy until it became virtually indistinguishable from ice cream. Did you know that a tiny tube of Go-Gurt squeezable yogurt has almost the same amount of sugar as a serving of Cocoa Pebbles? And most granola bars have even more sugar than both of those, yet we still put granola bars on a pedestal as a "healthy" food.

Sugar is addictive; some experts say it's just as addictive as cocaine. When we overeat sugar regularly, our brains create neural pathways that tell us that sugar is the route to happiness. We learn to associate sugar with pleasure, and of course we want more pleasure, so we reach for more sugar. The World Health Organization suggests that adults should consume no more than 5 percent of our calories from sugar, which translates to about 6 teaspoons per day total (both added sugars and naturally occurring sugars). For children, the recommended amount is about half that: 3 teaspoons per day, or 12 grams. The average American, however, eats 22 teaspoons (110 grams) of added sugar per day *beyond* the sugars naturally occurring in fruits and other foods. We're not even close to the recommended allowance—not even on the same scale.

I shudder to think about how much sugar Breanna and Nathan were consuming each day. I thought juice was healthy! It wasn't soda, and besides, it came in a friendly little box with a straw. Did I ever stop to read the label to find out that Capri Sun had 16 grams of sugar in each pouch? No. And if I had, it wouldn't have occurred to me that it was more than the entire recommended allotment of sugar for a day. After just one Capri Sun, Breanna shouldn't have had anything else containing sugar for twenty-four hours. Yeah, right! One Capri Sun and a granola bar for breakfast would have sounded skimpy to me, and yet it would have been more than three times the amount of sugar she was supposed to consume the entire day.

Surely no one ate that way, did they? I was convinced only the most obsessed health nuts could actually eat the way the experts told us to.

. . .

It was early 2011 when I told my sister how helpless I was feeling in regard to Breanna's weight. The whole thing felt like a losing battle. There were days when I knew I had to keep trying *something* or my daughter was going to live a lonely and possibly shortened existence, and there were other days I was too weary to fight and get my hopes up again.

"My niece lost twenty-five pounds in just a few months by joining a swimming club," my sister's boyfriend told us at a family dinner.

Swimming? The idea had potential. It wasn't as grueling as running the mile in gym class, and it wasn't hard on the joints. Breanna enjoyed swimming around in our backyard pool, even if she didn't know the right techniques. It was one of the few extracurricular sports we hadn't tried, and it made sense to me.

"Hey, Breanna!" I said the next day. "Do you want to join a swim club?"

She agreed—at least for the moment. There was a wonderful swim club nearby that I wanted her to join: Clovis Swim Club, one of the highest-ranked clubs in California. But I didn't want the coaches and other kids to see her the way she was and judge her. I thought it would be better to have her join a swimming club a little farther away and have her lose some weight first. Then, after she'd lost weight, I could transfer her to Clovis.

On the first day of swimming, it was difficult not to compare her when I saw the other girls jumping into the pool. While they moved with such ease, my daughter was a prisoner in her body.

They don't need help getting out of the bathtub, I thought.

The other parents and I sat on the benches and watched our kids splash across the pool. I couldn't help but wonder if any of the other parents had so much at stake. Was this the answer we were looking for?

Despite her limitations, Breanna was able to swim through the whole class. But predictably, as soon as the session was over and she was in the safety of my car, she said, "It's too hard. I don't want to go back."

I paused, considering my words. "Breanna, here's the thing.

I talked to Ryan, and he said that his niece lost twenty-five pounds in three months by joining a swimming club. I think you need to stick with this."

I watched closely for her reaction and saw a small glimmer in her eyes. What was it? Hope? Excitement? Fear?

"Okay," she agreed. "I'll do it."

I was elated. It was her first real commitment to any kind of physical activity in a long time, and it was a significant one—she'd be swimming five days a week. I wasn't looking forward to schlepping her back and forth for an hour in the car every day, but it was worth the effort if it would make a difference. I watched and waited, believing that if we just stuck to it this time, we would finally see results.

Even after we'd been there for months, we still felt like outsiders at times. No one told me what kind of swimsuit to buy for Breanna. I found out later, after asking other parents, that there were one-piece suits designed to help swimmers glide through the water with ease.

"The coaches didn't tell you what they recommend when you first got here?" one of the moms asked.

I shook my head, trying to believe it was just an oversight and not a slight. I noticed that they were teaching the other kids to dive, but they didn't teach Breanna. It seemed that they were just humoring us, not taking her seriously. They viewed the other new kids as future competitors, but not Breanna. She was just someone who paid tuition each month.

It did get easier for Breanna as the weeks went on. She didn't hate it, though she certainly didn't love it either. But at least she stopped fighting me about going.

Then one night, after she'd been swimming for about a month, I asked her to stand on the scale. I held my breath, my hopes soaring.

She'd gained more weight.

I wanted to cry. Well, I did cry, but not until she was out of sight. *How can she still be gaining weight? It breaks the laws of physics! God, this isn't fair.*

• • •

In the Bible study I attended through my church, we discussed Galatians 6:7: "Do not be deceived: God cannot be mocked. A man reaps what he sows." And 2 Corinthians 9:6, which says, "Remember this: Whoever sows sparingly will also reap sparingly, and whoever sows generously will also reap generously."

It is both a promise and a warning from God—what you do today affects your future. If you plant an apple tree, you can expect a bounty of apples. If you plant poison ivy, you can expect a pretty nasty rash. And it's important to know that you will reap *later* and *greater* than what you sow—it's not a one-for-one proposition. The results are not immediate, but you can expect them to be bigger than the seed you planted. That one apple tree can provide you with thousands of apples throughout its lifetime; that one poison ivy plant can spread across your lawn and infect everyone who passes through.

The same goes for the spiritual side of things. I had thought about how to sow seeds of faith. I'd tried to bring up my children to be kind and loving to others and obedient to God. But there were other seeds I'd been sowing all along too.

I had sown the seeds for obesity in my children without even realizing it, and now we were reaping. Boy, were we reaping.

We had sown by setting bad examples—eating junk—and by feeding them junk. We had sown by not setting proper limits and by being inconsistent in the ways we addressed eating and exercise. We had let them drop out of sports and live sedentary lives, and we had given in too many times when we said yes to a second or third helping to avoid listening to their begging.

God has provided us with all the food we need. It's right here, growing in the earth, and I was passing up God's provision and instead feeding my family things I could find in boxes and bags at the grocery store with dozens of unrecognizable ingredients and indefinite shelf lives. Some of that food could sit in a can longer than we would be alive—which isn't natural at all!

We'd sown by not educating ourselves better and by choosing not to stick to the principles the nutritionist taught us. We'd sown by expecting Breanna to follow a different set of rules from the rest of the family and telling her to eat healthy foods while the rest of us continued to eat whatever we wanted.

The harvest was daunting. I looked at my child, with her red cheeks and bunched-up skin, and my heart broke for her. I had no idea what it was like to live in that body, but it couldn't be easy. Every step was an effort.

Some days I went to bed thinking, *Tomorrow will be better. We'll figure this out.* And other days, I didn't believe that at all.

WHICH HAS MORE SUGAR?

One of the biggest challenges most of us face in eating healthy is not realizing how much sugar is in the foods we eat. Before we can successfully cut down on sugar intake, we have to know which foods are the culprits—and some of them may surprise you.

Here's a game you can play with your family as you learn together how much sugar is in common foods. You can continue playing with foods you find in your pantry and in the grocery store, and soon you'll be able to make more informed decisions about the foods you buy and eat. Try to guess which has more sugar.

1. Stonyfield Smooth & Creamy French vanilla yogurt vs. Kit Kat bars
2. Nature Valley Oats 'n Honey granola bar vs. Cocoa Pebbles
3. Minute Maid apple juice (8 ounces) vs. Coca-Cola (8 ounces)
4. Nesquick fat-free chocolate milk vs. Barq's root beer
5. Cinnabon cinnamon roll vs. Twinkie

Answers:

1. Stonyfield Smooth & Creamy French vanilla yogurt has more sugar (29 grams) than a package of Kit Kat bars (21 grams).
2. A Nature Valley Oats 'n Honey granola bar has more sugar (12 grams) than a serving of Cocoa Pebbles (11 grams).
3. Believe it or not, Coca-Cola and Minute Maid apple juice both have 26 grams of sugar!
4. Nesquick fat-free chocolate milk has more sugar (56 grams in 14 ounces) than Barq's root beer (50 grams in 14 ounces).

5. A Cinnabon cinnamon roll has way more sugar
    (59 grams) than a Twinkie (17 grams).

Tips for Cutting Sugar

Sugar is one of the biggest causes of obesity, and yet it's something people don't talk about the same way they talk about fats and carbs.

A great resource to help you get a visual idea of how much sugar various products contain is www.sugarstacks.com. It's one thing to read a label and see that something contains 20 grams of sugar but another to see what 20 grams of sugar actually looks like in the form of sugar cubes. It can be a shock!

Here are a few guidelines to help you start cutting back on sugar:

- Drink water or herbal tea before every meal. Drinking water has great benefits for weight loss—it has no calories, yet it fills you up and keeps your body hydrated and functioning properly. If your child complains that plain water is too boring, squeeze a little lemon juice in there. There are also endless flavors of herbal teas to choose from. You may think your kids would never drink tea, but you might be surprised. It's an acquired taste, and with enough exposure, they just might learn to like it.
- Forget sodas. Skip all sodas—even diet varieties, which are full of artificial sweeteners.
- Minimize juice. Apple juice has about 26 grams of sugar in an 8-ounce cup—exactly the same amount of sugar as 8 ounces of Coca-Cola! It's okay to serve juice every now and then as a treat, but pediatricians recommend no more than 4 ounces of juice per day, even for kids with a healthy weight. That's only half a cup. When you do serve juice, dilute it with water.

- Go for unsweetened iced tea. If you're ordering iced tea at a restaurant, you can't control how much sugar is in it. Go for the unsweetened kind instead. Also, make sure it's fresh-brewed and not from a mix.
- Ice cream and frozen yogurt should be reserved for very rare occasions. Believe it or not, low-fat frozen yogurt usually has more sugar than ice cream. If you eat a pint of it, you've just consumed twenty-two sugar cubes.
- Watch your sweeteners. It's common advice that if you want to eat healthy, you should substitute honey for sugar. But remember that honey is 80 percent sugar. A tablespoon of honey contains 17 grams of sugar—about the same as a Twinkie. Stevia has no calories or carbs, but it's still a new player as far as food additives go, and there haven't been long-term studies to show what the side effects might be. Agave nectar or syrup contains mostly fructose, and some experts think it is just as bad for you as high fructose corn syrup. Here's a better alternative: *stop trying to sweeten everything.* In time, your child's taste buds will adjust (and so will yours).
- Serve more veggies than fruits. Fruits contain natural sugars. A small amount of sugar is fine, but fruits and vegetables are not equal. Aim for a ratio of ¾ vegetables and ¼ fruits.
- Go for berries. Among fruits, berries are the best. They have a relatively low sugar content, and they also have fiber. Fiber is good for weight loss because it helps you feel full and flushes your digestive system faster. Raspberries are the big winners, with only 2.7 grams of sugar in half a cup. Blackberries and strawberries are close behind with 3.5 grams, and blueberries have 7.4 grams of sugar per half-cup serving.

- Use bananas as a natural sweetener. Bananas are great for you—but an average banana also contains 14.4 grams of sugar. Consider eating half of a banana and freezing the other half to be used later in a smoothie or to make your own "ice cream."
- Make your own. As often as possible, make your own food rather than buying prepackaged stuff—that way you can control how much sugar goes into something.
- Make substitutions. There are no perfect substitutes for sugar—basically, anything that makes things sweet either has a lot of sugar, a lot of chemicals, or an unknown safety profile. But even small reductions in sugar are helpful. If you're baking, substitute unsweetened applesauce for sugar. As a general rule, you can use the same amount of applesauce as you would have used of sugar, and then reduce the amount of liquids in the recipe a little bit to compensate.

CHAPTER 5

NEWS FLASH:
KIDS CAN BE CRUEL

EVERY TIME I GOT MY HOPES UP about the possibility of Breanna losing weight, they were dashed again. It felt so pointless—all the effort cajoling her into going to swim class, driving her back and forth, trying to make the schedule work with Nathan. Not only that, but she wasn't making any friends there. I made her keep going just because I knew that doing something was better than doing nothing, but I was almost resigned to the idea that Breanna would just be obese forever and there was nothing we could do to fix it.

My fears were growing about the social shunning she was starting to experience too. I knew that as she careened toward her teen years, things would get worse, not better. Every now and then she'd mention that someone was rude to her or that she knew other kids were getting together after school without her, but most days when I picked her up at the bus stop and asked her about her day, she was as stoic as ever, telling me that everything was fine. One day when she was in fourth grade, she finally told me there was a boy who was bothering her on the bus.

"You just tell me who he is, and I'll take care of it," I said.

"Don't say anything, Mom," she begged. "It'll just make it worse."

It was hard to rein myself in. I wanted to step in and fix things for her, but I held back. Until one day when she came home in major distress.

"He told me to pull down my skirt!" Breanna said.

"What?"

"On the bus. That's what he said: 'Pull down your skirt.' And then all the kids started laughing at me."

"Oh, honey. What did you do?"

"I said no, of course! Why on earth would I do that?"

I was irate. "I'm going to find his parents and talk to them."

"No, Mom, please don't. I don't want you to."

"Breanna, someone needs to tell this boy that he can't talk to you like that. I don't ever want him to bother you again."

"No, really. I'll handle it myself."

But the next day, things escalated. I was volunteering at school and went out with the kids at recess. Shortly after I got outside, Breanna told me that the same boy had hit her in the head with a basketball. I sent her in to the nurse's office to get an ice pack while the boy stood around with his friends, smugly claiming it was an accident.

I walked over to Breanna's teacher to talk about the

incident, and as I was standing beside her on the blacktop explaining what was going on, the boy and one of his friends walked by. His friend ran into me, bumping into me hard. As both of them walked away grinning, I had trouble believing this was just another "accident."

I went home that afternoon feeling angry on behalf of my little girl. And the worst of it was that I was only seeing the tip of the iceberg—the most visible acts. This boy and his friends had been tormenting my daughter almost every day. She regularly heard words like *fatty*, *ugly*, *fatso*, and *fathead* hurled in her direction.

In one of our more candid conversations, when Breanna was opening up about the bullying she'd experienced, I asked her about the first time she remembered being called names at school. She said it was when she was playing a game with a couple of friends on the playground and another girl came over to join in. After they'd been playing together for a while, out of the blue, the girl said, "Oh, you're chubby. You know you're chubby, right?"

"I don't know," Breanna said.

"You are. You're very chubby."

Her friends didn't say anything to stick up for her, and the girl made fun of her every day after that. Soon others joined in—both boys and girls, from her class and from grades above hers. They'd yell out insults while she was at recess—practically as soon as they walked through the door to go outside. Breanna didn't stand up for herself; she was too polite to tell them off and too timid to tell a teacher. So she took it every day and wondered over and over again why these kids were so mean to her.

• • •

Although Breanna had no real qualms about her body, she knew she couldn't keep up with the other kids, especially in gym class. Her biggest fear was running the mile for the Presidential Physical Fitness test each year. For two days ahead of time, she would be completely stressed out, begging to stay home from school, though we never let her.

But now the dreaded mile runs came on unannounced days. At least that meant she wasn't up all night worrying about it, but it caused her a lot of anxiety in school as she wondered which days she'd be expected to run the dreaded laps.

Inevitably, the faster kids would lap her, and she would finish last. She couldn't run for more than a few seconds at a time, so she would mostly walk. Afterward she was left feeling dizzy and nauseated and completely exhausted.

"Why can't I just call you to pick me up?" she'd ask me. "Why do we have to run? This has nothing to do with learning."

"I know you hate it, but just do your best. Exercise is good for you."

Yeah, right, she told me with her eyes. To Breanna, exercise was sheer torture. She liked most things about school; she dedicated herself to her schoolwork and projects, and that's where her self-esteem came from. When kids made fun of her, she'd remind herself that she was a good student, even if they could run faster than she could.

The kids who had been friendly toward Breanna in the earlier years were starting to find that it was becoming a liability to be her friend. If they hung around with her, they risked getting picked on too. There were only one or two girls who still talked to her and played with her at recess, but even they didn't say anything when other kids laughed at her and called her "Fatty."

One day a boy who sat behind her in class punched her in the back as hard as he could, and Breanna said nothing. The more the bullies got away with, the more their behavior escalated. She was the low girl on the social totem pole—the one whose worth was measured according to her weight instead of her character and personality. I'd always thought that if a kid was nice to other people, they would be nice to her. By that measure, everyone should have been nice to Breanna, because there was nothing mean about her. She always tried to be inclusive, even when others were excluding her.

Every year, we'd plan a big birthday party and invite all the girls in her class, plus everyone she knew from church— the more the merrier. One day she told a couple of girls at the bus stop that she was going to invite them to her party. They looked at her blankly.

"Yeah, the invitations are going in the mail soon," I added. "We'll make sure you both get one."

They glanced at each other and then back at me, straight faced. "We won't be able to go," one of them said. And then they turned and took a few steps away from us.

It was like being punched in the gut. I was so embarrassed; I couldn't imagine how my daughter must have felt.

"That was not nice," I said to the girls.

Then I turned to Bre. "Don't worry about them. Your family loves you and God loves you, and that's all that matters. It doesn't matter what those girls think."

She just nodded, and she never brought it up again. I found

out several months later that Breanna was already counting down the hours until the end of each day, waiting for the bus to drop her off so she could go into her room and cry.

When I think about that time now, it breaks me apart. I would give anything to have a do-over, to go back in time and set my kids up for healthy relationships with food and exercise. In addition to making life a whole lot easier for them physically, it would have saved Breanna from years of social torment and depression. But I can't go back. I can only move forward.

• • •

I knew Breanna wanted Dan and me to stay out of the situation with the boy who was bullying her, but we couldn't just let her be taken advantage of. After unsuccessfully trying to make progress with the boy's family, we decided it was time to take the issue to the school administrator. After three days of calling and a long weekend without hearing anything, I was finally able to schedule a meeting with the principal. This was a man I admired, and so did Breanna, and we hoped there would be a swift resolution.

Dan and I went to the meeting together, and things started out just fine.

"I'm glad to meet with you," the principal said. "I care about all my students as if they're my own, so I'm here to listen to whatever you have to say."

"We're having a problem with a boy who rides Breanna's bus," I said.

"Yes, I know all about it. He and his grandfather were in here earlier."

I was surprised, but I continued. "It started on the bus, and then the other day he hit her on the head with a basketball so hard that she had to have an ice pack on her head for forty-five minutes."

"I'm sure it was an accident," the principal said.

Dan and I were dumbfounded. Was he really going to dismiss the incident just like that?

"This wasn't an accident," Dan said.

"I know this boy," the principal said. "He's a nice boy from a nice family, and he's on the football team. I think you're seeing this wrong. I'm sure he didn't mean to hurt her. She was probably just in the wrong place at the wrong time."

"I think he's acting like a bully," I said. "And he's putting my daughter's safety at stake."

"If you feel that your daughter's safety is in jeopardy, you can always homeschool her."

I could hardly believe this was coming from the school principal.

"She doesn't want to leave school," I explained. "Why should she have to pay for something that someone else did?"

We spent almost half an hour in the office trying to convince the principal to do something, anything, to hold the boy accountable. Eventually we realized it was pointless to continue arguing, so we stood up to leave.

We'd heard stories about the administration siding with bullies before, especially when the bullies were star athletes or from well-to-do parents who made donations to the school, but this was our first time seeing it up close, and it was heartbreaking. How could anyone side with the aggressor?

But I also understood that it's easier to blame the victim

(who's usually more passive and agreeable) than it is to contact the bully's parents, set an appropriate punishment, and put monitoring in place to make sure the behavior doesn't continue or escalate. Often, instead of moving or inconveniencing the bully, schools will uproot the victim instead.

We could have tried to fight it out or take measures ourselves to ensure that the boy wasn't allowed near Breanna again, but we didn't want to fight an uphill battle that may not have had the desired effect anyway. Instead, I made sure Breanna never rode the bus again. For the rest of the year, we drove her to and from school every day.

It was a relief for both Breanna and me. She didn't have to hide who she was or try to disappear when she was in my car. I couldn't wait until the end of the year, when the bully would go off to junior high school and not be able to bother Breanna anymore. She still had two more years of primary school left, and I wanted her to be able to finish them in peace.

At the time, I thought this boy was the only problem. I didn't know there were many others like him who did less obvious things, like calling out ugly names as Breanna walked through the hall or laughing at her because of her weight. But I did know that my daughter was lonely and sad. It showed every day in her face, no matter what she did or didn't share with me.

We both loved the Taylor Swift song "The Best Day," a celebration of the mother-daughter relationship that talks about how even when the girl's friends turned mean, and she had no one to sit with in school, she knew her mother would take her on a drive and get her away from it all—until she "forgot all their names" and just got caught up in a great day with her mom. The lyrics fit what I saw with Breanna: the rare occasion when I saw some spark left in her was when we were away from home.

We'd take trips here and there or go out of town to visit family, and it seemed she was more at ease away from her home turf, without the weight of depression that followed her the rest of the time. I wanted the carefree Breanna to stick around, but we always had to get back to reality too quickly, and it wasn't long before the familiar shade went over her eyes once again.

God, I just want to protect my daughter, I prayed. *Why is this so hard? Please help her lose weight. Please help her fit in.*

I knew he was listening. But it was harder than ever to wait for an answer.

• • •

Going shopping with your daughter for her first training bra is supposed to be a sweet mother-daughter bonding experience. It's not supposed to happen when she's eight years old. But of course, things are different when your child is overweight.

It was becoming clear that Breanna needed a bra, so I took her to a store. We quickly discovered that there was no way she was going to fit into the dainty little things meant for preteens and teenagers. I had to take her to a women's store to try on bras meant for plus-size adults. We found some that would fit her cup size but none that would fit her band size. We ended up having to buy extenders to attach to the backs.

It's not cute or normal to see your third grader in a bra. Puberty—and all it entails—is not something you want to accompany playing with dolls and watching PBS Kids. The other girls her age weren't developing yet, and it made me realize that this was just one more thing that would make her an easy target for bullies.

Countless studies have made the connection between childhood obesity and early puberty, though researchers don't know exactly why. Obesity is not the only cause, but it's definitely linked with earlier development, whereas being underweight is associated with later puberty. Early puberty carries risks too: it usually comes with a growth spurt but causes girls to stop growing earlier than average because of the accelerated bone growth. So while an overweight girl may be taller than her peers at first, she'll wind up being shorter in the long run. Early development can also cause a lot of stress and social pressure for girls, and there may be an increased risk for breast cancer (so far, studies are inconclusive on this point).

Another problem is that it's hard to tell whether an obese girl is actually developing early or if she just has extra fat around her breasts. Doctors can't always distinguish between fat and breast tissue (and of course, neither can kids on the playground). So I was left waiting and wondering. Would her menstrual period start soon? I prayed that it wouldn't. She was my little girl. I reminded myself that things happen according to the Lord's timing, not mine, but even so, it felt like it was way too early for this kind of thing.

Please, God, don't let this be happening yet. She needs to be a child for as long as she can.

CHECKLIST TO IDENTIFY SIGNS OF BULLYING

If your child is being bullied, he or she might not tell you about it right away—whether because of fear, shame, or embarrassment. The Mayo Clinic offers some warning signs to look for:[7]

- ❑ Does your child come home with destroyed or missing electronics or other personal belongings?
- ❑ Does your child come home with ripped clothes or other signs of physical fighting?
- ❑ Has your child experienced an abrupt loss of friends?
- ❑ Does your child avoid talking about school?
- ❑ Does your child suddenly want to avoid social situations or school events?
- ❑ Does your child want to be left alone?
- ❑ Have your child's friends stopping coming around the house?
- ❑ Does your child try to skip lunch or recess?
- ❑ Is your child struggling in school, or are his or her grades declining?
- ❑ Does your child fake illness to get out of going to school?
- ❑ Does your child talk about hating school or ask to be homeschooled?
- ❑ Does your child experience outbursts of emotion (crying, anger) that you can't explain?
- ❑ Does your child complain about stress-related symptoms, such as headaches or stomachaches?
- ❑ Does your child have trouble sleeping or have frequent nightmares?
- ❑ Have you noticed a change in your child's eating habits?
- ❑ Does your child try to make himself or herself invisible (for example, by hiding in his or her room or wearing plain clothing)?

❑ Does your child seem distressed after spending time online or on his or her phone?

❑ Have you noticed your child withdrawing from friends and family?

❑ Does your child express feelings of helplessness or low self-esteem?

❑ Does your child exhibit shame about his or her body?

❑ Does your child engage in self-destructive behavior, such as running away from home?

What You Can Do

If you find that your child is being bullied, whether because of weight or other issues, here are some practical steps you can take.[8]

• Encourage your child to share his or her concerns with you.

• Find out the details of the bullying—how and when it occurs and who is involved.

• Ask your child what you can do to help him or her feel safe.

• Teach your child how to respond. For example, your child might try telling the bully to leave him or her alone, walking away to avoid the bully, ignoring the bully, or asking a teacher or other adult for help.

• Talk to your child about technology. Make sure you know how your child is using the Internet, social media platforms, or his or her phone to interact with others.

• Encourage your child to build friendships and get involved in activities that emphasize his or her strengths and talents.

• If necessary, contact your child's principal, teacher, or

school guidance counselor. Report cyberbullying to web
and cell phone service providers and websites.
- Look into a service to boost parental controls and
  monitoring for your child's Internet and cell phone
  activity. These sites may be good places to start:
    - http://www.socialshield.com (for social networking)
    - http://www.mymobilewatchdog.com (for smartphones)
    - http://www.spybubble.com (for smartphones, iPad,
      and Android tablets)
    - http://www.teensafe.com (for iPhones)

CHAPTER 6

180

In fourth grade, Breanna weighed 186 pounds and was round all over. I'll never forget one day when she accidentally stepped on my foot. It jolted me—I was shocked by how heavy she was. My daughter was carrying that weight around every day, and she could never set it down.

Although the sleep apnea hadn't returned, it sounded like there was a storm blazing through Breanna's room every night. *That can't be healthy*, I thought as I heard her wheezy breathing. But I certainly didn't want to take her in for another surgery.

She continued swimming at the club that whole school year. She was definitely making improvements, but she still wasn't being taken seriously. And she didn't really have any friendships to speak of. She'd attended the local Awana ministry for three years, but she hadn't bonded with anyone there, either. It stung to realize that even "church people" have trouble seeing past someone's exterior. At night, unbeknownst to me, Breanna would pray to God to make kids leave her alone in school.

After I dropped Breanna off at school, I would continue researching online, typing various phrases into search engines to see where they'd lead me.

childhood obesity
weight loss for kids
medical conditions causing all-day hunger in kids
plan to help a child lose weight
success stories of childhood obesity
before and after photos for children's weight loss
formula for children's weight loss
fitness programs for kids

I was constantly looking for the elusive answer I was sure was out there somewhere. It was easy to find success stories about adults who had lost weight and beaten obesity, but stories about children were practically nonexistent. The only thing I kept coming back to was that one weight-loss summer camp. There was nothing else—no support groups, no kid-appropriate diets, no exercise plans, no gyms for kids. Weight Watchers and Jenny Craig didn't have a "kids' division."

I found plenty of advice about dealing with obesity—*Cut out carbs! Exercise more! Stick to one thousand calories a day!*—but a lot of the advice was contradictory, and I still hadn't found a solid plan to follow. I didn't want random pieces of advice; I wanted someone to spell out a formula for me. Cook this; don't cook that. Do this kind of exercise X number of days per week and this other exercise Y number of days per week. If the plan came with specific targets to hit, even better. And I was desperate for ideas about how to overcome the biggest problem of all: my daughter's staunch opposition.

Along the way, I ran into some other scary discoveries, like the story of an obese eight-year-old who was taken away from his family by the Department of Children and Family Services. DCFS said they'd been working with the mother for a year to get her to help her child lose weight, but there had been no improvement. She was a substitute elementary school teacher who was also taking vocational classes, and she said that she just couldn't monitor him all the time, and that other family members sometimes gave him junk food without her permission.

A year after DCFS got involved, the boy was put into foster care. His mother was allowed to see him for only two hours each week. I thought about the time I'd basically checked out of Breanna's life when I was so sick during my pregnancy with Nathan. I certainly

Contributing Factors to Childhood Obesity

Thanks to a combination of factors, the current generation of children is by far the most obese. The obesity rate for kids ages six to eleven has quadrupled since the early 1970s and has tripled among kids ages twelve to nineteen. Not only are our foods more processed and filled with sugar and "supersized," but we also have a very different culture in terms of activity levels.

Kids today spend an average of seven and a half hours *per day* in front of a screen (television, computer, tablet, smartphone, video game). Only one in three kids is physically active every day. We adults aren't doing much better, either. Only about half of us report doing at least thirty minutes of exercise three times a week.

wasn't closely monitoring her food intake then. I could hardly believe she could have been taken away from me for that.

I kept reading and found out that as a third grader, the boy weighed 218 pounds. I swallowed hard—Breanna was getting awfully close to that number. If she kept up her current weight gain, it would be only another year and a half before she hit 218.

It's rare for children to be taken from their parents as a result of weight issues, but it does happen, both in the United States and in other countries. Just recently, two experts on childhood obesity from Harvard wrote a paper for the *Journal of the American Medical Association* encouraging the state to step in more often when kids are "severely obese" (having BMIs at or higher than the 99th percentile). They blamed childhood obesity primarily on poor parenting and said that in most cases, it was comparable to the effects of secondhand smoke on children.

The report went on to say that severely obese kids are at high (almost certain) risk of type 2 diabetes, which usually becomes permanent several years after its onset, and their life expectancies are cut short pretty significantly. Bariatric surgery is becoming more common, but at what cost? No one knows yet what the long-term implications will be for adolescents who undergo gastric bypass surgery, and there have already been cases of teens dying after the surgery. As a result, the report argued that instead of bariatric surgery, "placement of the severely obese child under protective custody warrants discussion."[9]

This revelation was terrifying to me. If I couldn't get Breanna to lose weight, the state could *take her away*? And from what I'd read, the tip could come from anywhere: a neighbor, a church member, a doctor—anyone could report us to DCFS, and from there we'd face an uncertain future. I shuddered to think that keeping Breanna in our house might be tied to the numbers on the scale—numbers that had never shown a sign of cooperating with our efforts. With the abusive households out there that still somehow had children in them despite evidence of abuse, could someone really take away my child for being too overweight and put her in a foster home with strangers?

The walls seemed to close in on me, and the air got heavier as I let the information sink in. Was it really all my fault that my daughter was heavy? Maybe I *was* a bad parent, as the researchers suggested.

These were the thoughts that plagued me whenever I was alone, and the ones that kept me up at night. I had nothing to comfort me except Jesus' words.

Mark 5:25-28 tells the story of a woman who needed God's intervention in a big way: "A woman was there who had been subject to bleeding for twelve years. She had suffered a great deal under the care of many doctors and had spent all she had, yet instead of getting better she grew worse. When she heard about Jesus, she came up behind him in the crowd and touched his cloak, because she thought, 'If I just touch his clothes, I will be healed.'"

One day I found myself on the couch crying out in pain to Jesus. I had been bleeding for many years too—not physically, but emotionally. I had taken Breanna to all the doctors, and her problem had just gotten worse. Now I just wanted to touch Jesus' clothes and have him heal my daughter.

"Why didn't you pick a mother like Kerry for Breanna?" I prayed. "She would know what to do."

Kerry was a good friend of mine whose son had been in Breanna's class in preschool. She was really into health and fitness, and she had trained her kids to say no to junk food without complaint. They willingly ate fruits and vegetables instead of doughnuts and cake. I was sure she knew a hundred recipes for healthy foods, and she always seemed to have her act together in a way that I did not.

"She even raises chickens!" I reminded God. "Her kids would never be in this mess. That's the kind of mother Breanna needs. I have no idea what I'm doing here."

I didn't hear a response from God that day, or the next. But a few months later, it came loud and clear.

• • •

A new family moved in across the street, and we liked them right away. Andrea and I had spoken a few times and exchanged phone numbers, and one day while I was on the computer in the midst of one of my down-the-rabbit-hole searches, she called and asked, "Would you like to go on a walk with me?"

Aside from a few walks our family had taken around the neighborhood, I wasn't much of a walker. But Andrea said she'd found a nice path and was hoping to find a walking buddy.

"Sure," I said. "Just let me put on some sneakers."

I had no idea that this was a moment that would change all of our lives. It was an ordinary weekday like any other. The "Hallelujah Chorus" was not trumpeting in the background, and no neon signs lit up to tell me that this was The Day. I wouldn't even know it was The Day until a couple of months later. But looking back now, it's obvious to me that this was where it all began.

Andrea met me at my door, and we headed out on a beautiful fall afternoon in California. Our town, Clovis, is in the middle of the San Joaquin Valley and is known as the Gateway to the Sierras. It's rich in Western culture and has a population of about 100,000. I'm sure it's always been a beautiful place, but all I knew of Clovis at the time was what I could see from the street: the shopping centers, grocery stores, movie theaters, schools, doctors' offices, restaurants, and hair salons. I had been all over the city by car and had seen the brick sidewalks and antique shops. I'd never walked anywhere beyond my own neighborhood before—but that was about to change.

Andrea and I walked from the back of my house along a canal that hooked up with the city's ten-mile trail system. Next to the path was a winding creek lined with majestic trees. The sun shone through the colorful leaves, and the breeze danced on my skin. The city was unbearably hot in the summertime, but now that it was fall, the weather was perfect.

This is Clovis? I asked myself. *I've been living here all this time, and I've never seen this?*

The view was gorgeous. It didn't feel like I was in my own city at all; I might as well have been on vacation somewhere— a place where people would pay to see views like this and get away from the hustle and bustle of normal life. I felt like I could breathe better out here, like the world had suddenly moved a little closer to heaven.

"Thank you," I said to Andrea when we got back home. "I never would have known about this if it weren't for you."

• • •

The company was as good as the scenery. Andrea had grown up in another country, and after her father abandoned them, her mother had left her in the care of her grandmother. They lived in a shack and cooked their meager meals over an open fire. Her life had been hard, yet she didn't seem to have any negativity inside her. She was a great mom who loved her kids and other people, and her stories were fascinating. I kept wanting to know more.

We walked and talked, and I lost track of time.

"Can you walk a little faster?" she asked.

"I'll try," I said. But I really couldn't. Andrea was taller than I was, which accounted for some of the difference, but mostly it was because she was in shape, and I wasn't even close. I might have been at a "healthy" weight, but that didn't mean much. My eating habits were atrocious, and I hadn't exercised since my school years, when I'd been forced to in gym class. Although I was enjoying the walk, it was physically hard on me. I hoped my friend wasn't too disappointed that her new walking partner was so slow.

We kept going, surrounded by still-blossoming flowers and twittering birds and a bubbling creek. When the walk was over, I was excited to hear her say, "Let's do this again soon."

I was sore the next day, to be sure, but I also felt enlivened. I told my family all about how beautiful our walk had been. Andrea and I went out several more times after that, and I learned that our route was a 3.8-mile loop. Not too bad! But shortly after we started walking, she got a job at a dermatologist's office, and our schedules no longer matched up. That was the end of our walks together—but I didn't want it to be the end of mine.

"You guys have to see this with me," I told my family one day in December. Fueled by my enthusiasm and the desire to see what I'd been talking about for weeks, they agreed to take the walk with me.

To be honest, I didn't think Breanna could finish the whole thing. It was a long walk, and I expected her to stop and sit down and maybe even cry at the side of the trail the way she'd done when she biked with my friend's daughter. At five, Nathan was overweight too, and I didn't know how long he'd hold out. But we took a leisurely pace, stopping to take in the beauty along the way.

To my delight, my family was just as enraptured by the scenery as I was, and we were able to finish the whole walk without disaster. Afterward we went back to the house, watched a movie, and ate a bowl full of buttery microwave popcorn, agreeing to do it again.

• • •

Every couple of days, on no particular schedule, we began walking together as a family. For the most part, I heard few complaints. Occasionally someone was tired or didn't feel like participating, but we did it anyway—"for the fresh air," I'd say. Breanna would stop and complain about her feet or legs hurting, but she didn't quit. And I was surprised that Nathan never balked at the distance. As it turned out, my kids were more physically capable than I realized. And not only was it a beautiful walk, but it also made for good family time.

When the kids were off for Christmas break, I decided to

keep up the walks. It was a better way to stave off boredom than sitting in front of a screen all day. We continued our walking into the New Year, even when it got a little chilly.

Honestly, I wasn't focused on weight loss at the time. I was just thinking that it was about time our family did something outdoors together, and I wanted them to enjoy the beauty around us.

One night in January after our walk, we went out to eat at the Spaghetti Factory. I'm not sure what possessed me to think of such a thing right after a big meal, but when we got home, I said, "Let's weigh in." I was so accustomed to these heart-sinking moments that the only question in my mind was, *How much has she gained?* Breanna never would have checked her weight if I didn't tell her to.

Breanna stepped on the scale.

It read 180.

She had lost six pounds.

• • •

Fireworks went off inside my brain. I let out a scream. Six pounds! I'd never seen the numbers on a scale go down when she weighed in—it had been a steady ascent of twenty pounds a year. And now, out of nowhere, six whole pounds were gone so quickly! I hugged her, hardly believing my eyes.

"Breanna! Look! You lost six pounds! This is so great! How do you feel? Oh, I bet this is because of the walking. It has to be because of the walking. This is just the start for you! Things are going to be different now!" The words kept tumbling out, falling all over themselves in a heap of joy and energy.

Breanna was nowhere near as excited as I was, but she

smiled anyway. I saw a little suspicion in her eyes, as if she were asking, *What do you mean, this is just the start and things will be different?* She was more than ready to go back to sitting on the couch.

But for me, the massive fog of confusion that had surrounded me for most of her life was suddenly dissipating, and something unexpected was coming into focus.

Hope.

For the first time, I realized we had a formula: swimming five days a week combined with frequent walks. Swimming alone hadn't been enough, but adding the extra walking had made a significant difference in just a few weeks. I couldn't believe it. All along, I'd thought that there must have been a more complicated answer than diet and exercise. There had to have been an underlying condition or bad genetics that was dooming her to a life of obesity. But the truth came barreling at me that day: exercise really did make a difference. And even better: walking was exercise! Who knew that exercise could be fun?

Sometimes you really can't see the forest for the trees, and I'd spent almost ten years staring at branches. Those six pounds on the scale could not be sending a clearer message. For the first time, I could see the forest.

In the movie *Soul Surfer*, professional athlete Bethany Hamilton says, "I don't need easy. I just need possible."

That's what we finally had: confirmation that this goal was possible. Breanna could lose weight. We had a long way to go, and I was under no delusion that it was going to be easy. But this was the first time I was going to lose sleep not because I was worried sick for my daughter but because I was too excited to rest. We finally had "possible." God had answered my prayers just in time.

HOW MUCH ACTIVITY DO YOU NEED?

Not long ago, the Department of Health and Human Services put out a set of guidelines for physical activity for Americans. Here's what they recommended for kids ages six to seventeen:

> Children and adolescents should get 60 minutes or more of physical activity daily. Most of the 60 or more minutes a day should be either moderate- or vigorous-intensity aerobic physical activity, and should include vigorous-intensity physical activity at least three days a week. As part of their 60 or more minutes of daily physical activity, children and adolescents should include muscle- and bone-strengthening physical activity at least three days of the week.[10]

And this guideline is just to *maintain* a healthy weight. Kids who are overweight and are trying to slim down need even more exercise than that.

Here are some activities that qualify as aerobic activity:*

Moderate Aerobic Activities	Vigorous Aerobic Activities
brisk walking (4 miles per hour)	jogging or running
water aerobics	riding a bike at a fast speed (except downhill, which doesn't count!)
playing volleyball	swimming laps continuously

* *Aerobic* means "requiring air." The term refers to any exercise that gets your heart rate up and your lungs pumping. You can tell the difference between moderate and vigorous activity by how hard you're breathing. If you can talk but not sing, it's probably moderate activity. If you can't say more than a few words without having to take a breath, it's vigorous activity.

Moderate Aerobic Activities	Vigorous Aerobic Activities
riding a bike at a moderate speed, on level ground	water polo
playing doubles tennis	using an elliptical machine at a vigorous pace
moderate dancing	climbing stairs at a vigorous pace
playing Frisbee	playing competitive basketball
shoveling snow	cross-country skiing
gymnastics	jumping rope
Muscle- and Bone-Strengthening Activities	
push-ups	squat thrusts
sit-ups	biking
gymnastics	

Tips for Fitting Exercise into Your Schedule

- If it sounds daunting for your child to do sixty minutes of moderate or vigorous aerobic activity all in one shot, break it up into smaller increments until your child builds the endurance to do a full hour.
- Make exercise part of your routine. Have your child do jumping jacks and jog around the block or backyard a few times, then jump on a trampoline, and later you can ride bikes together.
- Keep up the activity regularly. Exercising once or twice a week won't do enough to build up endurance; you want to get your child moving as much as possible every day.
- An added benefit to vigorous activities and muscle-building activities is that they speed up the metabolism. That means you're burning more calories even when you're not exercising!
- Getting started is as simple as going for a walk. Whether it's around your neighborhood, on a track, on a treadmill, or around the mall, just do it.

CHAPTER 7

RESISTANCE TRAINING

My poor family. They were about to meet an entirely different wife and mother from the one they'd known before.

The hope I experienced on the day I discovered my daughter had lost six pounds changed me fundamentally. It was a 180 in my life as well as on the scale. Never again would I be the permissive, easygoing mother who allowed my kids to finish off a bag of chips in one sitting or let them get away with eating two desserts at a dinner party. In an instant, I turned into Military Mom.

The day I saw "possible" was the day I realized we were going to war against nine years of bad habits. It was a war we needed to win, because my daughter's life was literally on the line. If we continued on our old path, it was clear what was going to happen to her: multiple health problems leading to an early grave, and a limited life where she wouldn't be able to enjoy the things other people can do with ease. Up until that day, I had almost resigned myself to accepting that fate. But now everything looked different.

It was the winter of Breanna's fourth-grade year, and I was determined that she was going to end this school year in a different place than where she'd started. To accomplish that, I needed a whole new mind-set to guide my daughter down the right path.

Before my breakthrough, the walks had been just for fun, whenever we felt like it. Now they were required parts of our routine, and the leisurely pace was over. If I was going to help my daughter turn her life around, we were going to do it wholeheartedly. My new plan was to walk as fast as I could and expect her to keep up with me.

I called it my "five, four, three" plan. Swimming five days a week, walking four days a week, and eating three healthy meals a day. I knew how to take her to swimming, and I knew how to walk the trail. But where I got tripped up was the three healthy meals part. It occurred to me that I didn't know how to cook a single healthy meal.

Not knowing where else to turn, I looked to the "experts." I bought frozen dinners from diet companies at the grocery store, and I took the kids to Subway for lunch when they weren't in school. *If Jared could lose all that weight eating at Subway, it must be good food*, I thought. The commercials showing Jared posing with his old giant pants were convincing. I wondered if Breanna would one day be able to fit herself into one of her current pant legs too.

Looking back, I can laugh at myself, because I know that

frozen dinners are not the answer. And now, just a few years into our journey, I can easily whip up dozens of healthful meals that take almost no time to prepare. But the important thing was that I didn't let my lack of knowledge stop us from making a start.

That's one thing I've learned along the way: you just start. You dig in and start somewhere, and then as you learn more, you revise your plan and fix your mistakes—but you start. Don't wait until you have the perfect plan; just take a step toward doing better than before. That's how real change is made.

* * *

The junk food was gone for good this time. No more locking it up, hiding it away, or tossing it out only to rebuy it a week later. I had to accept that if I was going to save my child's life, then I needed to set the example. I couldn't expect Breanna to behave differently from the rest of the family or to set limits on herself. We were the parents, and we needed to be the ones to set boundaries and stick by them.

Thankfully, Dan and I were on the same page. He was happy to see me get rid of the junk food for real this time, and he felt good about Breanna losing some weight. But there were also some tensions that surfaced almost immediately.

"Keep up with me, Breanna!" I would say when we were walking. Her dad held her hand, and they lagged behind Nathan and me. I had severely underestimated my son—he was usually the one up front, jogging ahead of the rest of us.

"I can't keep up!" Breanna would complain. "You're going too fast!"

"No, I'm not. Keep moving. You can do this."

"I need a break."

"There are no breaks," I said. "We're walking as fast as we can from the start to the finish."

"My legs hurt!"

"That's okay. Keep walking anyway."

"Heidi, give her a break," Dan finally said. "This isn't the Olympics."

I shot him a look that said, *Be quiet.*

Breanna could sense he was softening, and she started appealing directly to him.

"She needs a break," he told me.

"No, she needs to keep walking."

Over the next month and a half, we fell into a routine. Four days a week, no matter the weather and no matter what other conflicts came up, we went on our walk, and we went at my pace, period. But Dan kept insisting that I was being too tough.

He had a point—some of her complaints were real. Her thighs were rubbed raw and bleeding because of the chafing. She pointed to her legs, pleading for us to turn back.

"That's okay," I said without making eye contact. I knew that if I looked at my daughter, I'd give in. I hated to see her suffering, but I also believed this was for her good. "You're okay. We'll put some medicine on it when we get home."

This is temporary, I told myself. *She'll lose the weight and this won't be an issue anymore. Don't show sympathy, or she'll see an escape.*

When Dan and I were alone, we had some intense conversations about my approach.

"You're going too fast for her," Dan said.

"I'm saving her life. It's working."

"I think you're pushing too hard. She's going to start resenting you."

But I knew without a doubt that I was finally doing the right thing. In the big picture, what was too hard was having a daughter who wouldn't be able to breathe or run or do the things other kids could do. What was too hard was having my daughter get bullied and teased. What was too hard was watching as my daughter died a slow death, while I did nothing to stop it. *That* was hard. This was just a walk!

"You know what?" I said finally. "I love her enough to let her hate me."

I had never stood up to my children this way before—when they begged, I typically gave in. Now my resolve was being tested. Breanna was begging to stop the walks, and each time she came up with endless excuses about why she needed to stop. There was a pebble in her shoe. Her shoelace had come untied. Her shirt was itchy. She was hot and dizzy, and she was definitely going to throw up, and a bug flew in her shirt, and a twig was stuck in her shoe, and there was bubble gum stuck to the street, and it looked like rain was coming, and she was sure she was going to die of thirst, and she was sure her kneecap was going to pop right off. Some of those things were true, and some of them weren't. It didn't really matter.

"Keep going," I said. I wasn't going to waver. No matter what.

It was like a drug or alcohol intervention. Professionals in the field say that when you're dealing with an addict, everyone close to that person has to agree to follow the rules, and no one can stray from the plan. Many times, when an intervention fails, it's because someone on the support team caves. Someone gives in and hands the addict money or offers a place to stay or bails the person out when everyone had agreed not to. It's not that the support person wants the addict to fail; it's just a case of misguided sympathy. It's done with good intentions, but those intentions get manipulated into something harmful. The problem is prolonged, and sometimes people die as a result.

Our problem had been put off long enough; what I was looking at here was a nine-year-old whose childhood was already half over before it had really begun.

Obviously, our daughter was not a drug or alcohol addict, but she was addicted to food—and I was learning that this addiction could turn out to be just as deadly. Dan was taking her side not because he wanted my plan to fail or because he thought she was fine at her current weight, but because he was more concerned about her feelings than her obesity. But her feelings had led the way long enough. Now it was time for action.

"I think it would be better if you didn't come with us anymore," I said to Dan that night.

"What?"

"You're supporting her complaints, and I really feel like we need to show a united front. I need her 100 percent with me if this is going to work. I'm sorry, but I think it's for the best. I've been too soft in the past, and I don't want to make the same mistake again."

The next day was a whole new world for Breanna. She

didn't have anyone to complain to, and no one was going to stand up against me if she had some kind of pseudo-emergency on the trail.

"It's not fair! Why doesn't Dad have to go, but we do?"

"This is for your good, Breanna. It's helping you change your life and lose weight."

"I don't care if I'm fat! I'm fine being fat!"

"No, you're not."

"Yes, I am!"

"The way your feet hurt and your legs hurt, the way you have trouble breathing—that's all coming from the extra weight. When that weight is gone, you're going to feel so much better."

"I don't care."

"This is not up for discussion. We're doing the walk, end of story!"

She complained every few steps, but she kept walking.

As soon as we got home, Breanna stormed to her room while I went to figure out which dinners to microwave that night. We had a fine array of Lean Cuisine, Weight Watchers, and Healthy Choice awaiting us. Not exactly down-home cooking, but it was enough to keep us from starving. The kids didn't seem to mind the frozen dinners. Dan didn't care for them, but he didn't say anything. He knew I wasn't going to waver.

At the dinner table, I tried to tell Breanna about what life was going to be like when she lost weight. I set a goal for her: 130 pounds. She had no vision whatsoever of what it would feel like to be agile and energetic; to her, movement was the enemy. She couldn't imagine the idea of moving freely and actually liking it. To her, those athletic girls who lapped her during the mile were crazy for enjoying exercise. She didn't understand that some people could walk without their stomach rolls bouncing up and down, without their thighs rubbing each other raw, and without their feet developing painful blisters. She had never experienced "normal," so it was up to me to help her see it.

No matter how much I described this utopia, though, she wasn't buying it. But despite her protests, I didn't believe for one minute that she didn't care about being overweight. I knew my girl wasn't happy with her weight. She just didn't want to do the hard work that would fix the problem.

. . .

It would have been worlds easier to give in to the complaints and say, "Okay, you're right. Let's take it easy and just go for little walks every now and then when you feel like it." And Breanna might even have lost a little bit of weight that way, but that wasn't what I had in mind anymore. I wasn't looking for a ten- or twenty-pound weight loss. My goal was much bigger: I didn't just want my daughter to escape from the world of severe obesity; I wanted her to achieve a healthy weight and learn to live a healthy lifestyle. Nothing was going to stand in my way this time—not her, not my husband, not me.

I had to rely on God when I was met with resistance, and over and over he gave me the assurance I needed. I could sense him telling me, *You're doing the right thing. Everything will be okay.*

I felt my faith growing stronger as I handed my worries

to him. After all, he was a lot more qualified to handle them than I was.

The hardest part was figuring out how hard to push Breanna. Sometimes she would tell me that she felt like she was going to throw up, and I'd just say, "Okay, if you need to throw up, there's a bush over there." It never actually happened, but I promised myself that if it did, I wouldn't coddle her. I didn't let her stop for anything. I trusted that if there was a real medical need, I would be able to tell. It felt like God had instilled in me a heart of pure determination and a sense of confidence that we were finally headed in the right direction. I was not a bad parent; it had just taken me a while to get things figured out. I was a work in progress, just like all of us are.

I also took comfort in knowing that God had chosen me to be Breanna's mother, even when he could have chosen someone else. And if he had chosen me, then I knew he would equip me with whatever I needed to fight this battle. I didn't know what the next month or even the next week would hold; all I knew was that we had to keep putting one foot in front of the other.

We began weighing in once a week. In short order, Breanna lost another four pounds—bringing her to ten pounds overall. Ten pounds felt like a significant number to me.

"Look at this," I said, handing her a sack of potatoes. "This is what ten pounds feels like. This is the amount of weight you're not carrying around with you anymore. This is the amount of weight you never have to carry with you again."

The slightest grin crept onto Breanna's face. She didn't have to say anything. I knew that for the first time, this was starting to become real to her. Ten pounds of extra weight off her knees, her feet, her back. Every joint would work just a little better; every movement would be a little easier.

That didn't mean Breanna was fully on board. She no longer fought going to swimming, but she was ready to quit walking. It was one thing when our walks were something new, and we went at a leisurely pace, but having to exert energy and get her heart pumping felt like torture for her—not so different from running the mile for physical education. The scenery wasn't enough to keep her motivated anymore. Now it was just *work*.

I could have continued on like that, dragging her out to exercise against her will. After all, Dan and I were the ones who dressed her, fed her, put a roof over her head, paid for her school supplies, and gave her birthday parties. We were in charge of her physical and emotional well-being, and we hadn't done the best job living up to that responsibility until this point. But I also realized that this would go a lot smoother if I could find a way for Breanna to buy into our plan. At this point, the intrinsic reward of weight loss itself just wasn't enough for her.

So Dan and I came up with a new idea to motivate her. For every five pounds she lost, she'd get a manicure. For every ten pounds, she'd get an American Girl doll.

Yes, they cost a bajillion dollars. Yes, we were aware that if she were going to lose a significant amount of weight, then we were going to fork over a lot of money for dolls she probably wouldn't care about in a year. But she cared about them now, which was why she nearly fainted with joy when I told her that she'd just earned her first one.

Emily had gingery red hair and blue eyes, and Breanna loved her dearly.

Things got better for a little while after that.

• • •

When the kids had breaks from school, I tried to find active things for us to do as a family. During spring break we headed to Yosemite National Park for camping and a little hiking. I chose the Happy Isles trail because it was supposed to be beautiful and kid friendly. According to one online reviewer, "To walk the trails and bridges of Happy Isles is to commune with God and nature." That sounded good to me. I needed to recharge, and I suspected the rest of the family did too.

The hike was 1.6 miles round-trip and considered moderate in difficulty. A healthy individual—adult or child—should be able to complete it with relative ease. Yet Breanna was moaning and groaning as if she were climbing the Swiss Alps. She lagged behind the rest of us.

"Come on," I said. "You are not stopping!"

I hated to spoil the beauty of the hike by constantly badgering her to take each step, but it was the only thing we'd found that worked. Just like at home, she found excuses to stop every minute—rocks in her path, a bug in her face, anything. What should have been an enjoyable hike turned into a long exercise in frustration.

We had been camping a few times the year before the weight-loss journey began, after I'd seen a tent for sale at Costco and decided it was time to do something together as a family. The first time we'd gone camping was with my parents and my brother, and I was in charge of the food. We had sausage, bacon, and pancakes with maple syrup for breakfast; cheeseburgers, fries, and croissant sandwiches for lunch; steak with homemade French fries for dinner (I mean, who brings a bucket of Crisco on a camping trip?); and s'mores for dessert. I brought along my signature mayonnaise and my sour cream and onion chips, of course. In one of the pictures from another camping trip, Breanna is sitting with her hand in the marshmallows, eating them straight from the bag. That had been only a year ago, but a lot had changed since then.

When we got home and returned to our own regular walking trail, Breanna's complaints quieted for a few days, but her mood was still low. She asked if she could invite her friends on the walk because she was getting a bit lonely. She had one best friend and another fairly close friend, and we thought it was a great idea to have them come along.

Before long, though, things fell apart.

Breanna's friends were both thin and athletic, and they raced ahead of us. Breanna couldn't catch up, but they didn't seem to care. She was left in the dust, feeling like she did when she got lapped in gym class.

"Don't worry about them," I said. But Dan and I were disappointed too. There were so few kids who were nice to Breanna, and we didn't want her to lose them. But we didn't want her to be a doormat, either. Friends who leave you behind and make you feel bad about yourself aren't the kind of friends you want to invest in.

The next day, it was just us again. Breanna might not have been happy with me—she might not have even liked me very much at the time—but there was one thing she knew was true: I was never going to leave her behind.

WEIGHT-LOSS REWARDS

Many kids have grown up with food as their primary reward—and most often, unhealthy food. If your child isn't motivated by the idea of losing weight, then consider what kind of rewards might up the ante.

The long-term goal is for kids to have intrinsic motivation to choose a healthy lifestyle, but you'll most likely need to help them get there through external motivators, especially in the beginning. These rewards don't have to be expensive—the main thing is to figure out something that motivates your child. And eventually, someday, they'll learn that the best reward of all is a healthy life.

Here are a few ideas to get you started.

Tangible Rewards	Experiential Rewards
stuffed animals	beach
collector cards	amusement park
stickers	zoo
books	roller rink
dolls	bowling alley
games	movie
Privileges	concert
later bedtime on the weekends	"Mommy and me" day
day off from chores	"Daddy and me" day
music selection during family car rides	visit with cousins or other relatives
playdate or sleepover with a friend	
Monetary Rewards	
a dollar for every pound lost	

You can set small, medium, and final goals. I kept Breanna motivated by having a smaller reward she could earn about every three weeks (a manicure), a larger reward she could earn every other month (an American Girl doll), and a final reward (a big party with everyone she wanted to invite).

As you're thinking about rewards that would be meaningful for your child, here are some questions to consider:

- What things does your child love?
- How much money are you willing to spend?
- What things are meaningful to your child?
- What experiences have been significant to your child in the past?
- What privileges are meaningful to your child?

CHAPTER 8

TOUGH LOVE

THE MOST IMPORTANT CONCEPT in our weight-loss journey came in the form of three words that Breanna quickly grew to hate: *zero tolerance policy*. No excuses, no exceptions, no matter what. That policy was tested early on when weather conditions weren't optimal. People say things like, "You have to keep going through snow, sleet, or hail," but they don't really mean it literally. I did.

When I got serious about our walks, we were fully in the grip of winter. While we don't get snow in the Central Valley, it does get cold and foggy, making the early darkness of winter even more foreboding. Even so, we settled into a routine. I picked up Breanna from the bus stop and drove her thirty minutes across town to swim practice, and she ate a snack in the car on the way there. After our thirty-minute drive home, we immediately walked the 3.8 mile trail.

Sometimes the sky decided to mess with us.

"We can't walk today," Breanna would protest. "It's pouring!"

"That's okay. Your clothes will dry, and no one's going to drown."

Her mouth hung open as I handed her a raincoat. We walked in the dark; we walked in the rain; we walked in the hail. And we walked without umbrellas, because that would have just slowed us down. The trail was partly dirt, so when it rained, everything turned to mud and got slick. We walked anyway.

As the days got shorter and the sun set earlier, we walked in the dark. I felt some anxiety as a woman walking alone with two children, but I knew this was our ticket to health. So I carried a pocketknife as protection and pressed on.

We walked no matter what else was on the schedule that day. Four days a week our feet were pounding the trail, even if there was a school event, a birthday party, a dinner invitation, or a playdate. Those things would have to wait; the walks would not. They were mandatory, just like teeth brushing and homework.

I had to show my kids that I was serious. We weren't just aiming for minor change; we were starting a revolution! I wasn't shy about sharing our journey, either. While adults in weight-loss programs often have support groups to cheer each other on every time they lose a pound, we had to create our own support group. Every time we had a weigh-in and Breanna lost another couple of pounds, she would tell her fourth-grade teacher, who was enthusiastic and always encouraged her to keep up the good work. Her third-grade teacher would see her around school and make positive comments too. I shared the journey with my family and friends, especially the moms and teachers from Nathan's kindergarten class.

Breanna liked going with me in the mornings to drop him off. "I lost two more pounds!" she'd tell them.

The room would fill with choruses of "Atta girl!" and "Way to go!" as Breanna broke into a shy smile.

Not only was Breanna losing weight, but Nathan was too. When he was in kindergarten, he was seventy-six pounds and wearing size 10 husky pants. I thought that this was just his body type—that he took after his father. I didn't realize at the time that no one is destined to be overweight, regardless of what his or her parents look like.

By this time, I'd gotten accustomed to people's disapproving glances for having an overweight child. I was used to the stares and the tongue clicking when Breanna took a cupcake at a birthday party or finished off her juice box. At the mall, I was prepared for the sideways glances as we hunted for clothes that would accommodate her body. The judgment had been quiet, discreet. For the most part people conveyed their thoughts in their faces, not in their words.

But now I was experiencing a different kind of judgment. And this kind of judgment was something I'd never seen coming.

• • •

When we got serious about our plan, I decided that Breanna couldn't go to any friends' birthday parties. There were too many temptations: pizza, cake, cupcakes, goody bags, piñatas filled with candy . . . I didn't want to tell her that she couldn't have what all the other kids were having, so we just had her opt out. When the invitation came from a mother I knew, I would explain the reason, but that didn't always go well.

"Why can't she come to the party?" one mother asked me over the phone.

A Nationwide Epidemic

For the first time in history, the next generation of American children will have a shorter expected life span than their parents. According to studies by the World Health Organization, the average life span of people in the United States is nearly on par with developing countries. The average American now lives to be seventy-nine, whereas the average in Lebanon is eighty, Ireland and Germany are eighty-one, France and Luxembourg are eighty-two, Italy is eighty-three, and Japan is eighty-four.[*] Why are people in these other nations outliving us? A major clue is our diet and exercise habits. We eat junk, and we've gotten fatter and unhealthier as a result.

[*] "Global Health Observatory Data Repository," World Health Organization, http://apps.who.int/gho/data/node.main.688

"Because she just went to her cousin's birthday party yesterday, and she can't eat bad food two days in a row."

"What? It's my daughter's birthday, and you're not letting her go because she went to another party yesterday? That doesn't even make sense."

"She's been losing weight, but she still has a long way to go," I said. "I have to look out for her best interests."

"This is ridiculous. Next year, I'm not even inviting friends. We're just going to invite family, and that's it."

She hung up angrily.

To this woman, it was just one piece of cake at a party. To me, it was about teaching Breanna that the "kid culture" we were used to had to be limited. People who told me it was no big deal to let her have "just one" dessert didn't understand that it was like offering just one cigarette to someone who was trying to quit smoking. I hadn't endured weeks of complaints every few steps only to be thwarted by a My Little Pony buttercream cake.

I also encountered opposition when I turned down candy on Breanna's behalf. The same people who had judged me for letting her get fat were now judging me for sticking to a plan to help her lose weight. It felt like I couldn't win.

I wanted to tell people that if I continued being the soft mom I'd always been, my daughter would be on track to weigh three hundred pounds by the time she was in high school. I wanted to explain that an obese sixteen-year-old has a life expectancy that's thirteen years shorter than that of her peers. I wished I could tell them that if we kept up this pattern, there was a very real possibility that I'd bury my own daughter. I'd finally found a way to turn the tide, and no one was going to stand in my way.

God, help me endure this, I prayed. Sometimes it felt like every step on the walks was a prayer. *Help her to stop whining about her feet. Help her to understand why this matters. Please give us the energy to finish this walk. Help me to endure her complaints and her anger, and let other people's judgments bounce off me.*

I know for certain that the only reason I was able to be strong this time was because God was answering my prayers. He gave me a self-confidence I'd never had before. I didn't know exactly why our new plan was working, but it was. And I was able to face the challenges of each new day (often the same exhausting challenges over and over again) because I knew that the Lord was standing next to me, whispering in my ear that I was doing the right thing. This was his way, not my way. He didn't want my child to be obese any more than I did.

Truth be told, there were days when I didn't feel like going out either. Especially in the beginning, the walks were physically draining for me, too. My body had never been through real physical conditioning, and I was tired and achy and not thrilled about going out in the cold or the rain. And there were days in the beginning when I missed my Doritos and my comfort foods. But I never let my wavering show. I was the example, and I had to be strong for both of us.

One of the hardest things was telling Dan's mom that she couldn't bring her delicious desserts over to our house anymore. I knew it was her way of showing the family love, and I didn't want to hurt her feelings, but I also couldn't let the sugary treats tempt us anymore. I had to think of my kids and their future. We'd played footsie with obesity for nine years, and now the games were over. As soon as we walked in the door after swim practice, the orders were simple: "Put on your tennis shoes, and let's go."

That was all. Breanna could argue all she wanted, but she wouldn't get a rise out of me, and she wouldn't persuade me to relent.

The only thing that helped were the rewards. She looked forward to the manicures, but the American Girl dolls were the biggest motivation. When she stepped onto the scale, she had no reaction to the number she saw except as it related to moving her closer to the next reward.

The first pounds came off pretty easily for Breanna, as they do for most people who are significantly overweight. A lot of it was just water weight at first, but soon she hit more of a true pace. She wasn't going to earn a reward every couple of weeks, and that frustrated her.

One week the number on the scale hit 173, and I was

thrilled! Breanna wasn't, though, because it wasn't a reward number. She was down thirteen pounds total, but it would be two more weeks until the next manicure and seven more until the next American Girl doll. To a nine-year-old, that feels like a lifetime away.

She's eventually going to realize that being healthy is its own reward, right, Lord? I prayed. *Do you think maybe you could speed that part up?*

· · ·

On the weekends, Dan would occasionally join us again for the walks. On one of those days, our family was a mile into the walk when Breanna refused to take another step. She literally just stood there and refused to budge.

"Come on, Bre! Keep going!"

Nothing.

"It's just a walk. We've been doing this for a month already. You can do it. Get moving!"

"I am not moving. I am *not* moving."

I walked ahead of her. She stayed put. I yelled at her to catch up.

"My legs hurt," she shouted. "I am not walking anymore!"

I came unglued. "If you don't start walking again right this instant, I will take away all your privileges. Everything. I'm not kidding. You won't go anywhere, you won't do anything fun, you won't have any toys."

Dan and I did everything we could to motivate her to move.

"I don't care," she said.

Dan decided to head home with Nathan, and I asked him to remove Breanna's bedroom door when he got home.

I knew I couldn't physically drag her the remaining 2.8 miles. I couldn't pull a *Freaky Friday* and switch bodies with her for the rest of the walk. There was nothing else to do but turn back for home. On the way back, I told her that if she didn't get on board with this plan, she was headed for a lifetime of obesity and all the problems that came with it. She was quiet.

I told her about the problems and statistics I now knew by heart—how people with obesity face breathing problems, how they wind up needing surgery because of the extra weight on their bones and joints, how they experience higher rates of depression, how they have shortened life spans.

"Your decision to turn around and go home is a decision to choose diabetes and high blood pressure and heart disease."

She still didn't react. But when we got home, Breanna was in for a whole new world.

Dan had removed her bedroom door, taking away her beloved privacy. I herded up her dolls, including her American Girl doll, and removed them from her room, packing them away in a box. She sat on her bed silently as I did this, all the while telling her about the consequences of her actions. The most important one was this: "You're not going to Angela's house tonight."

All week, she'd been looking forward to going to her friend's house. They were going to have fireworks that night.

"No, you can't do that to me!"

"Yes, I can. The key to earning back your privileges is the workout. If you want to go to Angela's, you have to start that walk over again—and finish it this time."

She groaned.

"Breanna, listen to me." I was desperate for her to get it, and if I had to scare her in the process, maybe that was okay. "You're afraid of needles. Do you know what's going to happen to you if you don't lose weight? You're going to get diabetes. And do you know what happens when you have diabetes? You have to give yourself shots with a needle every day. Some people have to give themselves shots multiple times a day just to keep their insulin controlled. Your grandfather had diabetes, and it's a terrible disease. He went blind in one eye, and they had to give him a glass contact lens. Then he lost all the feeling in both of his legs below the knees because the blood wasn't flowing properly. They had to amputate one of his legs!"

I knew I was spilling out way more information than she needed, but once I started, it was like all my fears from the past several years poured out. "That's what obesity does to you. You don't understand it now, because none of this has happened to you yet, but it will if you don't change your habits now. Your grandfather never even got to meet Nathan. He died too young because of his diabetes—because he didn't take care of himself. He should still be here with us, watching his grandkids grow up. I'm terrified that something like this is going to happen to you."

I burst into tears, and so did she. These were not things I ever planned to tell my nine-year-old. I didn't want her to have to hear the gruesome details of what diabetes can do to you, but I was desperate. Maybe she needed to be scared if her attitude was ever going to change.

"You say that you don't care about your weight," I went on. "But I know you do. This body of yours isn't working the way it should. You've lost thirteen pounds, and that's an amazing accomplishment, but you still have a long way to go. That potato sack I handed you—you're still carrying around about six more of those that your body doesn't need. Your life could be so much easier if you'd just trust me on this. If we keep it up, you'll be able to move freely and run and jump. Nothing will get in your way anymore."

We looked at each other, tears streaming down our faces. There was still time to reverse this course. But it would have to be her choice.

"What do you want to do?" I asked.

She wiped away her tears, looked me square in the eyes, and said, "Mom, I have to finish the walk."

HOW TO CALCULATE BASAL METABOLIC RATE

Basal metabolic rate (BMR) is the rate at which we use energy when we're at rest. Even when we're sitting still or sleeping, our bodies are using energy—which means we're always burning calories. Weight gain occurs when we take in more calories than we burn. As we age, our BMR naturally slows down. It's important to do what we can to help kids increase their BMR so their bodies become more efficient at burning calories.

Use this link to calculate your child's approximate current BMR based on height, weight, and sex:

http://www.pediatriconcall.com/FORDOCTOR/pedcalc /basel_energy_expenditure.aspx www.pediatriconcall.com /FORDOCTOR/pedcalc/basel_energy_expenditure.aspx

There is no exact formula to determine how many calories your child needs to take in each day to live, but the USDA provides this chart as a guideline, including a daily limit for "empty calories" (snacks and drinks with no nutritional value):

Age and Gender	Daily Calorie Needs	Daily Limit for Empty Calories
Children 2–3 years	1,000 calories	135
Children 4–8 years	1,200–1,400 calories	120
Girls 9–13 years	1,600 calories	120
Boys 9–13 years	1,800 calories	160
Girls 14–18 years	1,800 calories	160
Boys 14–18 years	2,200 calories	265

Kids who are active need more calories than kids who are sedentary. Most kids have no problem figuring out if they're not getting enough calories—they get hungry! The bigger problem is figuring out when they're getting too many. If a child needs 1,400 calories a day but continually consumes 2,500 or more, that's going to result in ongoing weight gain.

BMR is partially genetic, but there are other factors that can influence it. Exercise burns calories not only while you're exercising but also for days afterward. And as you build lean muscle and burn fat, your BMR will increase as well, meaning that it gets easier to lose or maintain a lower weight as you go along.

CHAPTER 9

PLATEAUS, PEAKS, AND VALLEYS

I HAD NEVER FELT MORE PROUD OF or inspired by my daughter than I did at that moment. We headed right back out the door and did the full 3.8 miles. She didn't even complain about her legs or her feet. *Was this the turning point?* I wondered. *Will it stick?*

The answer was both yes and no. She never again stopped in the middle of a walk and refused to move, but this wasn't a "sunshine and rainbows" turnaround, either. She still had plenty of physical complaints. It was two more weeks before her thighs stopped bleeding. That was a relief for all of us, but even after that, she still had rashes and pain for some time.

I kept pushing harder; as I saw her fitness improve, I urged her to walk faster. She became tired of my rules and pushed back—especially on the "no birthday parties" rule. She couldn't stand being left out of other kids' parties.

"All right, then, we'll compromise. If you want to go to birthday parties, you can—within reason. Only one per weekend. But in return, you have to do the walk with me six days a week instead of four."

She rolled her eyes but agreed. "Fine."

One day Nathan had a doctor's appointment, and Breanna came with me. Then her pediatrician entered the room, and I said cheerfully, "Guess what? Breanna lost fifteen pounds!"

I expected congratulations. Instead we got a stern look.

"Well, don't let her lose more than sixteen pounds in a year. You'll stunt her growth."

How could he say that in front of Breanna when it had taken everything in my power just to get her to move? Did he not care that my 186-pound 9-year-old had just lost 15 pounds?

Breanna instantly turned to me and said, "Mom, I don't want to stunt my growth."

I was speechless. At the end of the appointment, he handed us gummy worms on our way out.

When we got into the car, I told Breanna, "Don't worry, honey. Losing weight isn't going to stunt your growth. We're going to continue what we're doing. You're doing great."

I was livid that a medical professional had discouraged her like that. And maybe he'd even put the smallest amount of doubt in my mind too. The next day, I called the weight-loss camp and asked them if it was true.

"No, it's not," the woman reassured me. "Do you have an older doctor?"

"Yes."

"Some of the older doctors still think that way, but multiple studies have disproven that theory. Losing weight definitely doesn't stunt kids' growth, no matter how much they lose, unless they're not getting the nutrients they need."

"Thank you." I exhaled, glad I could confidently reassure my daughter.

But now I couldn't stop blaming myself. Had this been my fault all along? Because of my own ignorance and the doctor's bad advice, I never realized that Breanna's weight problem was in my hands. I could have saved her from this if I'd understood from the beginning how to prepare healthy meals and make sure my kids got enough exercise.

It was hard to ignore the voice in my head that said, *This is all my fault.*

What could I do with a realization like that? Everything she'd gone through, from the surgery to the rashes to the inability to move to the social problems—all of it could have been avoided if I'd figured this out sooner.

Many nights my regrets drove me to tears. I wondered if I'd taken action in time for Breanna to experience a real childhood. So many wasted years were now behind us—years when other kids were busy making friends and joining sports. Would she still have time to develop those friendships and social skills that are so important? Or would my mistakes mean that she'd be disconnected from other people forever?

God doesn't shield us from every bit of guilt. We need to taste some of it so we can learn from our mistakes and become more empathetic. But when guilt is eating us alive and causing long-term pain, that's not from God.

I begged him to release me from my guilt, and he did. I will always regret that I didn't act sooner, but I have learned to move on. I know that if you don't, you'll stagnate right there and never take the meaningful actions necessary to fix the situation. In my case, I knew I was doing everything I could to correct the course, and I felt God gradually lift that burden from me. It's as if he was telling me, *You've repented and grieved. Now it's time to continue on the right path.*

• • •

On February 12, Breanna hit 169 pounds, and by March 5, she was down to 159. That meant another American Girl doll. As she saw the number on the scale, she jumped up and down. So did I—but for different reasons. Every time she stepped off the scale, I handed her something to show her what she had lost: ten-pound sacks of potatoes for the big numbers and pounds of hamburger meat for the individual pounds. I wanted this to be real to her. Now she'd lost two sacks of potatoes and was closing on the third, losing one to two pounds each week. The numbers on the scale weren't making dramatic drops from week to week as you see on reality shows, but there was steady progress.

During this time, the changes in Nathan's body were also undeniable. At age five he had weighed seventy-six pounds and was on the same obesity track as Breanna. For three and a half months, he'd been jogging ahead of us on the trail and eating the leaner foods we were eating as a family. In just that short span of time, Nathan had beat obesity. Not only was he getting remarkably fit, but the fat was vanishing. He would have an entirely different childhood from Breanna's.

He would never have to know what it's like to be teased about his weight or to feel isolated at school. And he would never have to fear gym class.

Things were going well . . . until Breanna's weight loss stalled. We were working out as hard as ever, but at her next weigh-in, she had actually gained a pound.

"That can't be right," I said. "It must just be water weight or something."

It took nine days for the scale to move again, and she was down only 1 pound—to 158. By the end of the month, she was at 157, meaning she'd lost only 2 pounds in the whole month. But she was also starting a growth spurt and building muscle, so despite what the scale said, her body looked healthier than before.

A pound of muscle has the same weight as a pound of fat. But it is also true that when you're building muscle, you may be losing fat even if you're not losing weight. She may have lost three more pounds of fat during that time but also gained three pounds of muscle, so they would cancel each other out on the scale. Also, since muscle is denser than fat, it looks different on the body—fat expands whereas muscle contracts.

There's more to weight loss than just the numbers on the scale, because lean muscle helps your body burn calories even in a resting state. A person with more lean muscle mass will burn more calories than a person with low muscle tone, even when they're both asleep!

Still, I wanted to see those numbers keep going down—for both of our sakes. After two weeks in a row of almost no progress toward her next goal, Breanna was disappointed.

So I decided we'd have to step up our game again. We were going to do something Breanna had never done voluntarily before: jog.

"No!" she said. "This is hard enough."

"Just three trees, Breanna. You see those trees up ahead? We're just going to jog to the third one."

"Ugh!"

But she did it.

Afterward she complained to Dan, waiting for him to back her up and agree that I was being unreasonable. Instead, he took one look at her and said, "Listen, you need to thank your mother for giving you a second chance at life. You don't realize it yet, but that's what this is. She's pushing you because this is the way you're going to escape a lifetime of weight problems."

It was a relief to know that Dan was behind me. He still didn't love my style, but he had learned to respect it.

I was coaching Breanna based on sheer instinct. I didn't know that what I was doing had a name and good science behind it: high-intensity interval training. That's the term for any kind of workout where you do brief bursts of aerobic activity followed by less intense activity. For us, jogging was very intense. It got our hearts pumping, and we both got winded fast. But it was exactly what we needed to add to the routine at that point, since this kind of training turns the body into a fat-burning machine. After an interval workout, your body continues burning fat and calories for twenty-four hours afterward. And the cool part is that you can work out for less time and get better results than if you didn't do those bursts of activity.

In the beginning, we just did a few bursts of jogging over the course of the 3.8 miles. Then, as we got stronger, we'd go a little farther with each interval. It was great to see Breanna rise to the challenge. She didn't like it, but she did it. I was so proud.

My daughter's metabolism had always been sluggish, to say the least. But as soon as we added jogging to the routine, her metabolism picked up, and we started seeing the numbers on the scale budge again.

"Mom! Mom!" she called from the bathtub one day.

I rushed over. "What is it?"

"Come here! Feel this."

She grabbed my hand and put it on her pinkie.

"You can feel a bone," she said.

She had never felt her finger bone before; it had always been padded in too much fat. It never even occurred to me that this would be a new sensation for her. There were so many little things I took for granted that she'd never experienced. I marveled with her—it was a magnificent bone, we decided.

• • •

That moment of discovery marked the first time that Breanna seemed impressed by the changes in her body. It was such a relief to me! Until that moment, only Dan and I had cared about what the extra weight was doing to her, but when she felt that bone, it seemed to set off a curiosity in her: *What else don't I know about my body?* If the lights had been out in her spirit before, now it was as if someone had installed a dimmer switch, and a glimmer was starting to return inside her.

As Breanna's confidence grew, she started taking more risks. One of the biggest was her decision to try out for the school cheerleading team. Although she gave it all her effort, she didn't make it, and she was devastated. We signed her up for a travel team outside of school instead—there were no tryouts for her age group, and anyone could join. I loved seeing my daughter in her cheerleading uniform with big bows in her hair. She was still bigger than the other girls, but I could finally see a future for her where that would no longer be the case.

Not long after she started cheerleading, we were walking on the trail one day when Breanna said, "There's a twig in my shoe!"

I was so used to hearing things like that from her that I just ignored her comment. But she repeated it twice more. "There's a twig in my shoe!"

"Fine," I said. "Stop and get it out."

"No," she replied. "I can't stop! I have to keep going."

I grinned. This was her way of letting me know that she was going to soldier on, just like I'd been teaching her.

While Breanna took baby steps on the trail, I was taking baby steps in the kitchen. It was time to move away from the frozen dinners every night, so I began asking everyone I knew about healthy cooking. Wherever I went, I picked people's brains about how to provide healthy options for my family.

The first lesson I learned was about frying foods. When I realized how unhealthy it was to prepare foods swimming in oil, I cut that out of our diet. Friends told me that protein and lean meats were important, so I tentatively cooked our first healthy meals: grilled chicken breast (the dark meat is too fatty), extra-lean ground beef, and a wide assortment of vegetables—prepared raw, cooked, and steamed in an attempt to find something the kids wouldn't hate.

For breakfast, Breanna would have a bowl of cereal. At first, she continued to eat school lunches, but after her weight plateaued for a second time, we examined our routine to see where we could make more changes. Though it took us months before we realized it, one of the most obvious changes was replacing the school lunch with a healthy, packed lunch. I hadn't paid much attention before to what most schools feed our kids—spaghetti and meatballs, fried mozzarella sticks, bagels and cream cheese, chocolate milk—almost none of it appropriate for a child trying to lose weight.

After school, she continued to have a rice cake and strawberries or blueberries as a snack, and then a healthy dinner. And for the first time ever, we enforced portion control. I responded to Breanna's complaints at the dinner table that she was still hungry the same way I responded to her complaints on the trail: with a firm "no."

Our new plan was still hard, but it was nowhere near as hard as it had been before I started seeing progress. Enduring the complaints is a lot easier when you see your child's clothes getting baggier. (I didn't mind the extra shopping when we were buying smaller sizes!)

Because I was so committed to this journey, and because I didn't want Breanna to feel alone, I did every workout with her. There wasn't a single step she took alone. After all, I wanted to be an example of not giving up. But after a while my own weight dipped into unhealthy territory in the other direction. It was an eye-opener for me to realize that I had to find a way to equalize the calories in, calories burned equation, so I increased my portions just enough. It wouldn't have done Breanna any good to have her mom collapsing in the middle of a jog.

Five months after we started our journey, just before the end of the school year, Breanna was down to 149 pounds. She was a different girl from the one who'd started fourth grade.

"You know the kid who punched me in the back?" Breanna asked me one day. "He looked at me today and said, 'Have you been losing weight?'"

"What did you say?"

"I didn't know what to say, so I just said thank you."

I was awed by the sight of her at thirty-seven pounds lighter. Her jawbone emerged, and her neck started taking shape. Some of the rolls disappeared entirely. Her thighs and calves had definition they'd never had before. Her breathing at night no longer sounded like a freight train. And beyond all that, she had a new self-confidence. Her posture changed; she stopped looking down when she entered a room. She started smiling again.

"She's coming back to us," I said to Dan, through tears. "She's coming back."

• • •

In her Bible study *Breaking Free*, Beth Moore gives a simple explanation for what happens when you're trying to break free from the bondage of something that's unhealthy—in our case, obesity. It looks like this:

hard ⇨ hardest ⇨ easier ⇨ under my feet

I was beginning to experience the truth of that cycle. Getting started was hard, but it was also fresh and new, so Breanna hadn't resisted as much on our first few walks. Then, when the newness wore off and it became work, it got harder. The first thirty-seven pounds were the hardest. Once she started noticing the results and liking how it felt, we moved to the next part of the cycle. It was easier now. I still had a hard time envisioning what it would be like to have the problem "under our feet," but I was hopeful we'd get there!

We set a new goal weight of 115 pounds. That was squarely in the middle of the healthy range for Breanna's height, and it felt like the right number. It was quite ambitious, considering she still had another 34 pounds to lose, but goals aren't really worth having if they're not big and audacious.

"When you get down to your goal weight, we'll have a party, and you can invite everyone you want," I told her. She liked that idea.

It made me giddy to even imagine we could do this. We'd come so far in less than six months; could it really take just a year to turn my daughter's life around entirely? I didn't even know what to envision for her anymore—before, whenever I'd thought about her future, I'd seen a picture in my mind of a woman who could barely move, someone who was reclusive and shy. Now I felt as if I was getting to know my child all over again. *This* Breanna was more like the one I'd known in preschool and kindergarten, only more grown up. She was the one who danced in the living room with wild abandon. That's who I saw tentatively peeking out now, and it made me so happy.

She could do anything with her life, I thought. *There won't be any limits.*

The more she lost, the more she was found.

HOW MANY CALORIES CAN YOU BURN IN THIRTY MINUTES?

If you're feeling stuck in a hard spot right now, keep in mind that even thirty minutes of activity here and there can make a difference in your child's metabolism, muscle building, and overall health. The chart below gives you an estimate of how many calories people can burn, depending on their weight, in thirty minutes of each exercise.[†] For more information, you can go to http://www.healthstatus.com/calculate/cbc.

Activity	125-pound person	155-pound person	185-pound person
basketball	240	298	355
bicycling	240	298	355
cross-country skiing	240	298	355
dancing	180	223	266
downhill skiing	180	223	266
elliptical machine	270	335	400
football	240	298	355
gardening	135	167	200
gymnastics	120	149	178
high-impact aerobics	210	260	311
hiking	180	223	266
hockey	240	298	355
horseback riding	120	149	178
ice skating	210	260	311

† "Calories Burned in 30 Minutes for People of Three Different Weights," Harvard Health Publications, Harvard Medical School, http://www.health.harvard.edu/newsweek/Calories-burned-in-30-minutes-of-leisure-and-routine-activities.htm.

Activity	125-pound person	155-pound person	185-pound person
jumping rope	300	372	444
kayaking	150	186	222
low-impact aerobics	165	205	244
martial arts (judo, karate, kickboxing)	300	372	444
mowing the lawn (powered push mower)	135	167	200
raking the lawn	120	149	178
rollerblading	210	260	311
rowing machine	210	260	311
running (12 minutes/mile)	240	298	355
shoveling snow	180	223	266
skateboarding	150	186	222
ski machine	285	353	422
sledding	210	260	311
snowshoeing	240	298	355
soccer	210	260	311
softball	150	186	222
stair-step machine	180	223	266
stationary bicycle	210	260	311
step aerobics	210	260	311
swimming	180	223	266
tennis	210	260	311
volleyball	90	112	133
walking (17 minutes/mile)	120	149	178
water polo	300	372	444
water skiing	180	223	266
weeding	139	172	205
weight lifting	90	112	133
wrestling	180	223	266

CHAPTER 10

SO THIS IS WHAT IT'S LIKE TO BE HEALTHY

It wasn't all smooth sailing after that, though. When the school year ended, as relieved as I was for some reasons—I didn't have to worry as much about bullying anymore, for one thing—I was terrified for one main reason: summer would entirely disrupt our routine.

First was the problem of all that free time. When Breanna was in school, it meant that for most of the day, she didn't have the option of snacking. Now she'd be home much more—and she'd potentially be bored. How would I keep her out of the kitchen and away from the television? And then there was the even bigger problem: we weren't going to be able to continue our walks much longer.

In the Central Valley, June is the first of four months of unrelenting heat, and while I could make Breanna soldier on in the cold and rain, the heat was a different beast altogether. It was flat-out dangerous to exert ourselves in those temperatures. Local athletes are often up before the sun, getting in their workouts before the heat becomes too oppressive. And even then, it isn't uncommon for the temperature to hit eighty degrees and climbing fast by six o'clock. There isn't much I wouldn't do for my child, but none of us wanted to be out there on the trail before six in the morning.

Plus, the increased pace of our walks had reached the limit for Nathan's little legs. He was a trooper and jogged along with us, but he just couldn't go faster. I had asked neighbors and friends to watch him while Breanna and I walked, but I was stretching those resources thin. I needed a solution for the heat and for Nathan.

We went to the local health club a couple of times, and to my surprise, Breanna loved working out in the gym. She enjoyed the gym culture—the loud music, the buzz of activity, the collective energy of athletes in motion. The facility also had a two-story play structure in the child-care area that was just right for Nathan. It was the perfect solution!

Well, almost.

The glitch: Breanna wasn't old enough. The membership forms clearly stated that no children under the age of twelve were allowed to use the facility. I called all the other health clubs in Fresno County and was crushed to discover that none of them offered fitness equipment to children under the age of twelve, and sometimes even fourteen.

I had a serious moral crisis. While Breanna could easily pass for twelve years old, it went against everything in me to lie. Yet here I was with an obese daughter who had momentum on her side and who actually *wanted* to go to the gym. How could it be that in a country where one in three children is overweight, there were no gyms where kids could get real exercise?

I wish I could say that I talked to the owner and got permission. I did not. The fact is, we went to the gym and pretended Breanna was twelve. I had her memorize her new birth date and the grade she was allegedly going into, and I told her that she could never, ever tell the truth to anyone at the gym.

Jesus, please forgive me, I prayed. *I feel like I don't have much of a choice.*

Each time we walked by the reception desk, I had a moment of panic that we would be discovered, and our membership would be revoked. Later I found out that the owner of the gym would have made an exception for Breanna—he is a good man with a heart for kids battling obesity. But I was so afraid of being kicked out at the time that I didn't dare risk it.

When we first started at the gym, I knew nothing about gym culture. I didn't even bring earbuds or headphones for us to listen to music on the treadmills, so Breanna and I just talked. It was good mother-daughter bonding. The best part of the treadmill for me was that it took away my need to nag Breanna to keep up the pace. When you're on a treadmill, it's a fixed speed—if you don't keep up the pace, you fall off! So I was able to walk on the machine next to her and talk to her instead of constantly calling out, "Walk faster!"

There were days when we got to the gym and I would realize that I'd forgotten my running shoes. Much to Breanna's amusement, I ran barefoot! There were days when I had a pulled hamstring, and once when I had a hideous chest infection, but I made myself continue to move, no matter what. Then there was a time when Breanna had a broken arm and couldn't swim or run, so instead we increased the incline on the treadmill and walked faster.

There will always be something to hold us back, because that's just life. I never made an excuse to quit, because I didn't want to set a bad example for Breanna. I either did the workout or had Dan do it in my place. I treated our times at the gym like they were a matter of life and death, because they were. No matter what life threw at us, we went to the gym.

We set the treadmill pace at four miles per hour, and I was thrilled with how automated the process became. We could walk for five minutes and then jog for five minutes, alternating between the two. As the weeks went by, we increased our speed. Before long we were legitimately running for twenty-five minutes out of our hour and fifteen minutes on the treadmill.

After a while, I bought Breanna an iPod, and I started using my phone to listen to music. We found that music was a great motivator. I left the music off during the walking and then turned it on just when we started jogging so I'd have something to look forward to. Breanna also liked watching YouTube videos during the workouts.

A few weeks into our gym routine, Breanna spotted her back in the mirror when she was wearing a tank top.

"Look, Mom!" she said. "Look at my shoulder blades!"

She had never seen her shoulder blades before. For that matter, *I* had never seen her shoulder blades before.

"Can you take a picture so I can see them better?" she asked. It was a big moment for both of us. I still have the picture.

• • •

In June, I felt that Breanna was ready to switch to the Clovis swim club. While I was at it, I signed up Nathan, too. I noticed a difference immediately; the instructors treated her as an athlete right from the start. They were serious about teaching her and turning her into a competitor. She would go through their summer program as a new member and then join the regular team in September.

I was grateful to see that the coaches taught her how to dive right away. As I watched the practices, I was surprised to see that there were other overweight kids there doing the same things she was doing. It made me realize that I could have started her at that club in the first place, and they wouldn't have been judgmental the way I'd expected.

The kids seemed nice, but I didn't see Breanna approaching anyone or trying to make friends there. I hoped that would change, but I didn't push the issue—I was nagging her enough as it was.

It was a serious time commitment to have my kids involved in all these activities, but it was worth it. Nathan took to the water easily, and I began to see the possibility that Breanna could be a really good swimmer someday.

Can my kids actually become athletic? I wondered. It was a thought that would have seemed laughable a year earlier, when they were both wasting the day away watching television and eating junk food. But now just about anything seemed possible.

. . .

We stuck with Jared and his Subway for lunch every day. *Every day!* I know. But that's the thing about progress: you can't tackle everything at the same time, or it's too over-whelming. So much of my time was now spent going to the gym, bringing the kids to their activities, and doing research. I was beginning to feel confident cooking us dinner each night, and breakfast was simple enough to get out of a box, but I didn't trust myself enough to cook two meals a day. So we stuck to the whole wheat bread six-inch subs—usually turkey with lettuce and cheese, and no soda or chips.

For fun, my kids loved going to a big indoor trampoline facility in our area filled with trampolines, foam pits, monkey bars, obstacle courses, and a dodgeball section. Even better, they had a $49 pass for the whole summer. It was perfect— the kids saw it as fun, and I saw it as a workout. It became part of our routine nearly every day. My only rule was that they were to be jumping the whole time we were there—no standing around.

More and more, we found ways to incorporate exercise into our daily lives, even beyond the walking and swimming. Gone were the days of sitting around in our air-conditioned house watching television; now we were up and moving for most of the day. Every weekday, Breanna got three separate workouts: the gym, the trampoline place, and swimming. After a few weeks, I decided to change it up a bit with a summer pass to the local water park on Fridays—another kid-friendly destination that inherently required motion. (I was surprised how tired I was after a day of dragging rafts and climbing stairs to the top of slides!) I quickly learned that we needed to pack a lunch on Fridays because there were no healthy options at the water park. It's amazing how unhealthy the options are at most "kid-friendly" places! No wonder kids eat such lousy food—it's what they're conditioned to like.

We had a blast that summer as we learned the joy of physical activity. In some ways, I was developing a unique brand of cross-training, as each workout (treadmill, trampoline, waterslides) used different sets of muscles. It was a wholly different lifestyle, and to our surprise, we were actually learning to enjoy it.

. . .

Up until this point, I hadn't known how unhealthy I was. Because I was a normal weight, I'd never bothered about diet and exercise—I thought the only reason to care about those things was if you wanted to lose weight. Sure, I'd heard that exercise was good for you, but somehow I'd decided that didn't apply to me. But now I knew it was true. I had so much energy!

Getting out of bed and starting my day was significantly easier. I didn't feel like I needed a nap in the middle of the day. It was like being on a natural high all the time.

So this is what it's like to be healthy!

Without anyone having to tell me, I knew that what I was doing now was extending my life as well as Breanna's.

As for Bre, she had more energy too. She was usually the one who asked me to go to the trampoline place, which I couldn't even imagine her doing before. Whereas she used to sit still whenever she could, she willingly spent an hour jumping, climbing, and running all over the place with her little brother. She was discovering her body for the first time—testing its limits and seeing what it could do. She was still overweight, but she was much stronger and more flexible, and movement was no longer a negative thing. My prayers were being answered faster than I could keep track.

That summer I read an article in my local newspaper, the *Fresno Bee*, that angered me. It was the first time I could remember seeing my paper cover childhood obesity, and it was a shockingly negative article. The article was about the staggering effects of childhood obesity here in my hometown. It told the story of a young boy who was going in for surgery because his growth plates were being crushed by the excess weight he was carrying around. The article gave a rundown of scary statistics and described the horrible things that can happen to obese kids. For a day or two, I stewed about it, wondering if permanent damage had already been done to Breanna's body. It upset me to see so much negativity without a hopeful ending. Finally I decided I had to take action. *I have to call the writer and tell her the other side of the story.*

The journalist's phone number was included at the end of the article, so I called her and told her what it's like to be in the trenches of childhood obesity. I let her know how few success stories and role models were out there. I asked her if she'd write another article, and this time talk about the hopeful side of things—that obesity is treatable, curable, and preventable.

The journalist was respectful and interested in what I had to say, and she called me later to say that she wanted to feature Breanna's story in an article about kids in our area who were losing weight. I was thrilled with the idea, but I didn't know how Breanna would feel about it.

"Bre, there's a writer who would like to talk to you about your weight-loss journey and maybe put your picture in the paper. How would you feel about that?"

"Really?" she asked. "I think that would be so cool!"

"Even if the kids in school see it?"

"Yeah! Why not?"

I was so proud of her, and I told her that by being willing to tell her story, she could inspire a lot of other kids. The journalist and a photographer came with us one day to the trampoline place and chatted with us as the kids played.

"Look! I'm going to do a flip," Breanna called out. She

Genetics and Weight

Scientists are still at the beginning stages of understanding the link between genetics and weight. While there are genes associated with childhood obesity—at least nine of them that we know about so far—no child is destined for a life of obesity just because of their DNA. Yes, some kids are born with slower metabolisms, bigger appetites, or bodies that have difficulty burning fat. But that doesn't mean they have no hope—they just may have to work harder to avoid temptations and maintain a healthy weight.

In a way, obesity is similar to alcoholism. There are genetic components involved, but not everyone who is predisposed to alcoholism will succumb to it. In order to become an alcoholic, you have to choose to drink. If you never choose to take a drink, then your genes are irrelevant. Where obesity differs is that it's not an option to not eat. But as long as you're making healthy food choices and staying within your recommended daily calories, you will never be overweight, no matter how "doomed" your genetic profile may look.

jumped high in the air, did a flip, and landed on her feet with a big smile. It was hard to believe this was the same kid who hadn't been able to finish the mile run at school.

The article ran in August 2012. Breanna was featured along with three other local kids who were also making strides in their battles against obesity. The paper ran two photos of her. In one picture, she held her fourth-grade school photo, and the difference was shocking just from her headshot. The other photo was of her leaping in the air in a cheerleading split at the trampoline park, smiling broadly. This was the new Breanna.

The reaction from our friends, family, and community was so encouraging that I wondered if we should go further than our local paper.

Would anyone else be encouraged by her story? I wondered. I was so inspired by her that I wanted to let other parents and kids know that change was possible. I thought of all those times I'd felt so alone and lost, looking for success stories. Now here we were, creating our own.

I contacted CNN's hotline and told them about Breanna—how she'd already lost fifty-seven pounds in less than eight months just through better eating habits and exercise. A producer called me back and expressed interest, but then we played phone tag for a while, and eventually one or the other of us gave up. I was so focused on other things that I didn't think much more about it.

• • •

One of my ongoing concerns was to keep improving our eating habits. As I learned more, I made more adjustments to our food routine. A friend told me, "Don't drink your calories," and that led me to the decision to cut out juice altogether. We stuck to water—lots and lots of it! As a special treat at a restaurant, I would ask the waiter to blend a cup of ice and then put in just a splash of orange juice—our own form of healthier Slushees. Another friend said "fat equals fat," prompting me to pay attention to the fat and saturated fat content on nutrition labels. Another friend taught me about the vicious cycle of sugar cravings. Dr. Mark Hyman, a family physician and bestselling author, talks about how sugar is more addictive than illicit drugs. "The $1 trillion industrial food system is the biggest drug dealer around, responsible for contributing to tens of millions of deaths every year," he said in the *New York Daily News*.[11] And what's more, he explains, you can't exercise your way out of a bad diet.

I'd heard about the low-carb trend, so for a brief time, we significantly reduced Breanna's carb intake. But I discovered that she actually needed good carbohydrate sources to sustain her through her workouts.

For us, the bigger enemy was processed flour. We ran from anything with the word *enriched* on the label or anything that didn't contain the word *whole* (multigrain or wheat bread is not the same as whole-wheat bread!). We focused on true whole grains, such as whole-grain bread (whose first ingredient is "100 percent whole wheat"). We even decided to try sprouted whole-grain bread again, which the nutritionist had recommended when Breanna was in preschool. This time, surprisingly, it didn't gross us out. We had gotten used to whole grains by then, and it was no longer so strange to our palettes.

Once we switched over, we never switched back. Knowing

that sprouted bread is easier to digest, has more vitamins, and contains minerals that are easier to absorb, I felt really good about this choice. To my surprise, we didn't miss our old white bread at all—in fact, now white bread tastes weird to us.

I called the weight-loss camp again and decided that if I couldn't get Breanna into their camp, at least I could ask for some advice. I told them about our progress and how much exercise Breanna was getting. Then I asked if they could give me any tips about a meal plan.

"Well, here we focus on no more than twenty grams of fat per day and as little sugar as possible."

I adopted that as our official plan. I didn't want to count calories, but counting fat grams and looking out for sugar sounded doable. Over time, I stopped believing the hype on the front of packages and started understanding the labels on the back. I learned that you need some dietary fat to live. It's a vital part of building healthy cells, developing the brain, regulating hormones, and cushioning the organs. Without enough fat, your skin will be dry and your body will have trouble absorbing vitamins. But these are healthy fats we're talking about here (olive oil, eggs, avocados, and nuts)—not Cheetos.

We were nowhere near worrying about too little fat with Breanna. Twenty grams of fat per day was enough for her body to function well without giving her extra to store. I learned about shopping the perimeter of the grocery store: that's where the real foods, like produce, meats, and dairy, are found. It's in the inner aisles that you get into trouble with the packaged garbage loaded with preservatives, artificial sweeteners, and other assorted chemicals.

. . .

By the end of the summer, Breanna weighed 130 pounds. She had lost an additional eighteen pounds since the end of the school year. She still had more to lose, but she felt and looked like an entirely different person, even to herself.

"Mom, you're not going to believe this. I didn't recognize myself today."

"What do you mean?"

"I walked by a mirror and looked behind me, because I thought it was someone else."

She had the biggest grin on her face. She still had never admitted to me that she cared about being overweight, but there was no question she was excited about her new appearance. And we were both excited about our next excursion: to the mall.

It had been years since Breanna had worn anything other than T-shirts and elastic-waist skirts, while so many of the other girls her age shopped at Justice, a haven of glitter and animal prints and pink sequins and stylish sundresses. The last time Breanna had been there, she'd walked out in shame when she realized she couldn't fit into anything in the store. But not this time.

She went into the dressing room with a shirt, her face filled with hope. A few minutes later, she peeked out the door with a big smile. It fit! Breanna couldn't wait to show off her new look and tell her friends about the progress she'd made.

"I like the new me," she said.

Later that day, a mom we knew spotted Breanna. "You're looking good, Bre! I like your shirt."

"Thanks," she said. "It's from Justice's new collection, just released yesterday."

I got such a kick out of that. Overnight, she'd become a fashionista, and for the first time in years, I got to buy my girl cute clothes like I'd always dreamed.

We were all a little sad that summer was coming to an end, but for once I was excited about sending the kids back to school. I was so hopeful that Breanna would be treated differently this year, and that she would make some real friends.

Dan and I walked both kids onto campus that first day of school. It was Breanna's first day of fifth grade and Nathan's first day of first grade. We watched as she walked with her chin up and her shoulders back, radiating confidence and pride. What a contrast it was to the first day of fourth grade when, at 180 pounds and nearly bursting out of her skin, she had squeezed herself into a size 10½ wide shoe and a women's XXL shirt. Now she was down to a regular size 8 shoe (who knew shoe sizes shrink too when you lose weight?) and child's size 14 clothes. She didn't need a bra anymore, either.

I watched as she passed kids she knew and said a quick hello. Then I watched their expressions: *Is that Breanna?*

Breanna found some of her friends from the year before, and as they were all talking, a boy Breanna had known since first grade came up to them and asked, "Who's the new girl?"

He didn't even recognize her.

I gave her a hug good-bye, and as soon as I turned around, I cried tears of joy.

TIPS FOR EATING OUT

The best plan is to eat out only on rare occasions since there are so many temptations, and the portions at most restaurants are so large. And since restaurant food is almost always less healthful than what you can make at home, it's best to think of dining out as an occasional treat.

- Select the healthiest option available on the menu, and then split it with another person.
- Say no to French fries or chips as a side. Ask if you can have extra vegetables instead. If your child eats one serving of French fries, it accounts for his or her entire allotment for fat for the whole day, with no nutritional value!
- Ask for healthy substitutions whenever possible (for example, turkey bacon instead of regular bacon, whole-wheat bread or a wrap instead of white bread, fat-free dressing instead of creamy dressings).
- Ask the server not to bring a bread basket.
- Limit your drink options to the following: water, herbal tea (no sugar), or a cup of blended ice with a splash of juice added.
- Dessert is not an option unless you're ordering fresh fruit.
- Don't get suckered into something just because it's "included." Sure, a kids' meal might come with soda or juice and ice cream, but you can say no!
- If meals come in giant portions, ask the server to just bring half the meal so it's not sitting there on the table.
- Don't show up to a restaurant feeling ravenous. If you know you'll be going to a restaurant, eat a healthy snack before you go so you won't be tempted to eat too much.

CHAPTER 11

THE NEW KID

I HAD BEEN SO WORRIED FOR SUMMER to start and mess up our routine, but now I was equally worried for summer to end.

We had settled into a pattern that worked over the summer. With Breanna in school for most of the day, I'd have to relinquish some of my control. Now she'd be sitting down for about six hours straight every day, with minor breaks for recess and physical education. It wasn't that long ago that she'd been sneaking a second breakfast at school and canvassing the lunch table for leftovers.

"Please, God, be with her and help her make good decisions," I prayed. "Put good examples in her life, and help her to resist temptations."

Breanna had a wonderful teacher for fifth grade. I spoke to her about not allowing Breanna to have any candy, cupcakes, or cookies in class—whether for birthday celebrations or otherwise. She understood and said she was glad to make the accomodations necessary for Breanna during the school year. I also appreciated that her teacher didn't put up with any bullying. Although Breanna still wasn't making friends, it was an easier year for her socially, and there were fewer incidents of kids tormenting her.

In addition to all her other activities, Breanna joined the school basketball team and tried out for the school cheerleading squad for the following year. This time, with a year's worth of practice behind her, she made it. She was ecstatic!

With all of Breanna's after-school commitments, including longer swim practices from 5:30 to 7:00, it was getting more difficult to get to the gym. I decided it was time to make a significant investment in our family's health, so I bought two treadmills for our home. It was a lot of money—about $700 apiece—but it was also our assurance that we'd never have an excuse to miss a workout.

Having workout equipment at home meant that we could do part of our workouts in the morning before school. I wanted us to work out every day for one hour and fifteen minutes, and if there wasn't enough time to squeeze that in between school and swimming, we'd do part of the workout before school and part of it afterward.

Despite our routine, though, Breanna's weight loss slowed once school started up—and then we got a truly unpleasant surprise. In the two weeks around Halloween, she gained four pounds.

There was no great mystery here: Halloween parties were in full swing and the classroom was full of candy. I'd been getting a lot of flak from other parents about just letting her enjoy the holiday, and I let it get to me. I hadn't stopped her from partaking in "kid culture," and now we were paying the price. It made me realize that, left to her own devices, Breanna could wind up right back where she'd started. I had to shake things up, so I took away her final safety net.

"You are not holding on to those handrails anymore," I told her. She had always held on to the sides of the treadmill to keep her balance, but that was preventing her from getting a full workout.

"I have to! It's how I keep my balance!" she argued.

"You'll learn to balance without them."

She may not have liked it, but once she realized she could do the workout without holding on, she seemed to get an extra burst of determination. I felt like I was watching a race-horse with blinders on, finally focused on winning.

She lost the four pounds plus some, and then she zipped up her first pair of jeans.

"Mom, look!"

She still thought I was mean for making her go through all this. Yet whenever she ran to show me these "firsts," I knew we were sharing a bond that comes only from digging through the muck of adversity together. The difficulties made the rewards that much sweeter.

• • •

Now that the kids were in year-round swimming at Clovis Swim Club, Breanna began competing in meets. One of the best parts of the sport was that the competition really wasn't about beating someone else—it was about achieving your own personal best. The swimmers would support one another at the meets, and everyone would congratulate those who shaved off time in their event.

After a few months of this six-days-a-week swimming schedule, I was sitting on a bench one day when I saw a girl named Jacqueline come over to greet Breanna.

"Hey, Breanna!" she said. "How was your day?"

"Good, except I had a science test. It was really hard. How was yours?"

The interaction was so . . . normal. Except that it wasn't. It had been so long since I'd seen anyone come over and talk to my daughter like that—so long since someone had offered her friendship.

I could hardly believe it, but I was starting to see the spark in my daughter's eye again.

The swim club became a second home for Breanna. Not only was it a great place for her to train and compete, but it was also a tight-knit group where she made close friends. It started with Jacqueline, but soon Breanna had a whole group of friends from swimming who would come over to our house. I wondered if she'd be embarrassed to tell them her story or show them pictures of what she looked like before, but she wasn't at all shy. In fact, she was proud of how far she'd come.

We continued adding pieces of exercise equipment here and there until we had a full-fledged gym in the house. We opened it up to anyone who wanted to use it, which meant that we regularly had friends and neighbors coming by to work out with us. We invited them to join us on the trail, too. It was just what Breanna had craved when we'd started the walks.

These changes were also a sign of the emotional transformation that was happening inside Breanna even as her body was changing. Over the next few months, Breanna's whole personality began to blossom. There was a time when she never would have approached someone she didn't know well, but I watched in amazement as she became more outgoing and self-confident.

Kids began inviting her over to their homes, which was both great and scary. If she was out of my sight, I would have no control over what she ate, and I couldn't yet trust her to make the right decisions. If someone put out a plate of cookies or brownies, would she eat them? And if so, would she stop at one or two? Even though she was proud of herself for the weight she'd lost, you can't trust the willpower of a hungry ten-year-old.

I learned to ask the sometimes uncomfortable questions. When Breanna would ask if she could go over to a friend's house, I'd speak to the mother on the phone first.

"I'll feed her lunch first, so you don't need to worry about that," I'd say. "Do you know what you're giving them for a snack?"

If the answer was anything other than fruits and veggies, I'd say, "Okay, I'll send her with her own snack, because we're focusing on healthier eating habits."

My approach was always received well. Sometimes the mother would say, "Great. Send some extra, and my daughter will have fruit with her."

I loved that, because then Breanna didn't have to feel different. It felt like we were hitting a groove—both physically and relationally.

Then something terrible happened: Breanna broke her arm.

It happened during cheerleading practice. The girls were taking a water break, and Breanna wanted to see if she could do a back walkover—where you bend backward until you're upside down and then kick your legs over your head until you're in a standing position again. She fell onto her arm, and I had to rush her to the hospital.

I was terrified that her injury had something to do with the weight loss making her bones weak, but he said it had nothing to do with that.

"Is it because of a lack of calcium?" I shot the doctor a nervous look. "She never drinks milk. Can you do a bone density test?"

"We don't need to," he said, pointing to her X-ray. "Her bones look fine. This will heal, but she needs to take it easy for the next few weeks."

"What does 'take it easy' mean?"

"She can't get the cast wet. No running, no jumping. . . ."

I couldn't breathe. Six weeks of no swimming, running, cheerleading, or jumping? That was almost our entire exercise plan! The only thing left was walking. At least she was still allowed to do that. I wouldn't let all our progress be thwarted like this.

I had an idea: since we couldn't do our intervals of walking and running anymore, we would put the machine up to a 10 percent incline at intervals to take the place of the run. It was like walking up a steep hill. Breanna didn't like it, but it was the closest we could get to a real workout.

I was on edge for the entire six weeks. I didn't want to set us back on the weight loss, and I was afraid of what would happen if her arm didn't heal properly. Breanna didn't lose any weight during this time, but she didn't gain any, either. And when she went back to the doctor for the follow-up, he proclaimed that her bones had healed perfectly, and she was cleared to go back to her normal activities.

What a relief! That very day, we went back to business as usual. Back to swimming, back to running, and back to cheerleading . . . with the admonition not to do anything without a spotter again!

The best side effect of her injury was that we got to know some of the doctors and staff at Valley Children's Hospital. Not only were they wonderful to her, but they were also interested in her weight-loss story.

"You lost *how* much?" one of the doctors asked Breanna. "Do you know how inspiring that is? Do you know that you're a role model?"

That made us feel so good. The doctor told us that she dealt with so many kids who were struggling with their weight—many of them even dealing with diabetes. She asked if she could share Breanna's story with them so they would know that it was possible to be successful just through healthy eating and exercise. Of course we said yes! We felt great knowing that Breanna could help other kids see that there was hope.

• • •

In November I got an unexpected phone call. It was the CNN producer, and he wanted to run the story about Breanna after all.

"Sorry we fell out of touch," he said. "It just got crazy with election coverage. But we'd like to run an article about the two of you in the health section of our website."

We were excited to share our story with the world. We had lived with the effects of obesity for nine years, and if we could help even one family and let them know that obesity intervention works, then it would all be worth it.

When I woke up on the morning of December 4, I turned on my computer to see the article about Breanna's journey. To my surprise, there she was—one of the top new stories on CNN's website, right next to a picture of President Obama!

My heart raced as I clicked on the article. It was an honest, fair portrayal of what we'd been through. The piece quoted Dr. Denise Wilfley, director of the Weight Management and Eating Disorders program at Washington University School of Medicine, with her suggestions for combating childhood obesity. "Mainly what we suggest is actually having the whole family take on a healthier lifestyle—for everybody to eat as well as possible, as nutritiously as possible, so the overweight child is not singled out," she said.[12]

I thought back to the days when I would make corn on the cob and give everyone else their corn slathered in butter while Breanna's was plain, or when I'd make cold cuts sandwiches with mayo for everyone else while hers was on dry bread. I expected my daughter to get active, but I didn't participate in that except to drive her around and cheer her on from a chair.

That wasn't a reasonable expectation. "Do as I say and not as I do" is hypocrisy, and children can see right through it. If I wasn't willing to eat healthy or exercise, how could I expect my daughter to? We all had to get on board.

When CNN featured the article about Breanna, she weighed 121 pounds. She had dropped sixty-five pounds in just under a year, and she'd done it in a healthy, methodical way. She was just eleven pounds away from her goal weight. There was no question in either of our minds that she was happier and healthier than ever, with more energy, more friends, and more self-confidence than we had imagined possible.

That same day, HLN called, saying they wanted to do a Skype interview with Breanna and me. We were excited but nervous—it's not every day that you get to share about your journey on a national platform. *The more we share our story, the more parents and children we can encourage,* I thought. *People need to know that change can happen one step at a time.*

During our interview, Breanna opened up about how kids had made fun of her. She said, "I got teased almost every single day."

My heart broke for her all over again as I heard about the pain she'd endured for all those years.

A Real-Food Experiment

When I see people who have eating habits like we once did, I want to tell them, "Put down your cheeseburgers, fries, and sodas for two weeks. In the meantime, eat real produce, whole grains, and lean meats. At the end of the two weeks, try your fast food and unhealthy choices again. I guarantee it won't be appetizing anymore." After eating healthy foods for two weeks, you'll feel more alive than ever—you'll have more energy and be more alert. You'll realize the fog you were living in wasn't normal. Our food should give us energy to take on the world, not hold us back from it.

CNN ran several before-and-after photos with the article, and I was so proud of Breanna for having the courage to show them publicly. She never expressed concerns about the comments she might get or worried that kids might make fun of her. One of the "before" photos was of her in the pool in a bathing suit. Although she was clutching a kickboard, there really was no hiding what her body looked like. Looking at the picture now, I can't help but think that being obese is like being a prisoner in your own body.

Breanna enjoyed her newfound sense of celebrity, especially when the segment aired on CNN's HLN with Mike Galanos. The best part for me was receiving Facebook messages like these:

> Hi. I came across your story on CNN. I have a nine-year-old who is very overweight also. Our story sounds very much like yours. How did she lose the weight?? I'd love to know more. :)

> I'm sure you're being inundated with messages after the news story about your daughter, Breanna, but our family identified so much with your story! My daughter, Kate, is five years old and already dealing with obesity issues, and we are so frustrated.

> Hi Heidi. I watched your story of your daughter on CNN. I also have a nine-year-old daughter who is overweight. I would love to know more about what exactly you did. My heart breaks for my daughter every day at school, where she is faced with other kids' comments.

It was like I was in a time portal, speaking to myself a year earlier. I knew the pain behind these letters. Not long ago, I'd been in the same place, searching for answers, just as these people were now. It felt like an honor for Breanna and me to be able to help these people.

"Do you realize that you're an inspiration for children all over the world?" I asked her.

She nodded and gave me a big smile.

"What do you think we need to tell them?" I asked.

"That all you need is a pair of tennis shoes and motivation," she said. "Tell them that change can happen one step at a time, and it's worth it."

So that's what I told them. And then the craziness began.

• • •

It all started when we got calls from *The Biggest Loser* and *Good Morning America*. When the producers from *Good Morning America* called, they were ready for us to fly out to New York that day. I had no idea how to respond. We had work and school and sports and, of course, the workouts—which really were mandatory. Not even *Good Morning America* could get us to skip our exercise routine. We explained our predicament, and they offered to wait a day.

"We'll fly a crew out to visit you in California and follow you around," the producer said. "You don't have to change anything for us—we want to see your regular routine. They'll interview you and see Breanna in action at her different activities. Then we'll fly your family out to New York for the weekend. You can do some sightseeing, and then we'll do the segment on Monday morning."

We said yes and then did a little screaming. Within twenty-four hours, we had to figure out a wardrobe for the whole family that would be appropriate for a national television appearance, and we had to pack for New York. We could barely get our minds around the fact that we were going to be interviewed by George Stephanopoulos. How surreal. How intimidating. How exciting!

We'd never been to New York before, and there was no way we could possibly fit everything we wanted to see into one weekend. But we were certainly going to squeeze in as many adventures as we could.

As soon as we got there, I stocked our room with healthy food so we wouldn't be tempted by all the street vendors selling pretzels and hot dogs, or the luscious breakfast buffets. Fortunately, it wasn't hard to exercise in New York; it felt like the whole city was one giant walking club! We made our way around Manhattan on foot, joining the thousands of other locals and tourists doing the same thing. Afterward, we worked out at the hotel gym just as we did at our gym at home. We splurged a little on dinner because we wanted to sample the famed New York cuisine, but we were still careful about our portion sizes and didn't overdo anything.

Being on set at *Good Morning America* was both nerve-racking and wonderful. Everyone there was supportive and eager to celebrate our journey with us. Just as I'd hoped, Breanna's story was presented as a positive example for other parents whose kids were struggling with weight issues—a chance to see the human side of the childhood obesity epidemic.

George Stephanopoulos asked me how we did it, and I explained our exercise routine and our plan to eat twenty grams or less of fat per day and as little sugar as possible. Breanna felt really good about the appearance. Of course, we didn't tell Mr. Stephanopoulos what we'd done the day before the show. To me, this is one of the funniest parts of the story. Breanna was a huge fan of the show *Cake Boss*, so the night we arrived in New York, Dan looked up the address of Carlo's Bakery, which is featured on the show. He realized it was just a short trip from where we were staying, so we headed there the day before the interview.

It was a dream come true for Breanna. When we were there, the owner's sister was in the bakery mingling and talking to the customers. She came out to meet us, and I told her our story. She congratulated Breanna and gave us a private tour of the bakery, even serving us lobster tail pastries fresh out of the oven. This was an occasion that called for a once-in-a-blue-moon splurge!

• • •

The day after the *Good Morning America* show aired, we headed home. Though we'd loved visiting New York, I was happy to get back to our routine. Breanna still had eleven more pounds to lose before she hit her final goal.

That day when we were flying home, Breanna's teacher shared the segment about Breanna with the class. In the interview, Breanna talked about the mean nicknames she'd been called.

After the show ended, her teacher said, "We've all said or done things we wished we hadn't at times. I'm hoping that if any of you have said or done something that hurt Breanna's feelings, you'll think about apologizing. It may be hard, but it's the right thing to do."

Breanna never received any apologies.

That didn't seem to rattle her, but I hold out hope that maybe, as her story gets out there, it will prevent another kid from getting teased the way she did.

In the meantime, we continued to feel God at work in our lives. Both Breanna and I remembered what it was like to feel hopeless, and we were so glad to be able to help other people who were in the same spot we'd been in. If I thought I'd gotten a lot of positive feedback after the CNN article, that was nothing compared to what came in after *Good Morning America*.

Messages of support and requests for help came pouring in from all over the country and even the world. Just a year ago, I'd been paralyzed with fear about my daughter's future and consumed with hopelessness over not knowing how to help her. Now God was using me to encourage other people who were facing the same challenges I'd faced. I truly believe God opened these doors for us. Without him none of this would have been possible. He has helped us spread our message of hope because he cares about the health of all his children, and he desires for us to live to our full potential.

Here are a few of the messages I received:

I just finished watching your inspiring video on *Good Morning America*. I am the mother of two beautiful daughters, and I am very concerned about them. . . . We have had the same tests your daughter went through, and everything has come back normal. I was wondering if you could help me and my husband put our daughters on a healthier path. You and your daughter are an inspiration, and I am pleading to you as one mother to another.

I just watched the program on *Good Morning
America*. I couldn't help but just cry. I am dealing
with the same thing right now with my seven-year-
old. I was so moved and inspired. . . . Most of all
I felt hope.

One of the comments I enjoyed most came from the friend
of a friend. She said that the day after they saw the show, the
whole family bought new tennis shoes, since Breanna had
said that was all you needed to get started. They were eager
to start following our path.

I saw the needs of mothers who were dealing with their
children's weight problems. Breanna saw the needs of kids who
were dealing with depression and bullying. As we were faced
with these very real needs, I saw a deeper side to my daughter.

I'll never forget her response to someone who was thinking about suicide:

Killing yourself is not the answer. The people who
are bullying you do not care about you. They don't
care if you live or die. You aren't hurting them. It's
your family and the people who do love you who
will be hurt.

After Breanna's story aired, it went viral. It was covered
by Fox News as well as other news stations across the United
States. It showed up in thousands of web articles and blogs,
and ended up as a top trend on Yahoo and on the main
page of Bing. Her story reached as far as Mexico, Australia,
Britain, and Malaysia. Over the next couple of days, we got

calls from *The Doctors*, *The Steve Harvey Show*, and the *Today* show in Australia asking us to appear. It was mind boggling.

Each time a new article appeared, the Valley Children's Hospital staff would print it out and post it on the wall so other patients could see it. They were so proud!

But along with the positive feedback and the requests for help came some negative comments, too. Dan and I read some of the online comments, and I got a fast education about what a "hater" is. I never knew that there were people just lying in wait for a new bone to pick—anyone to criticize and tear apart. They said the craziest things—accusing me of making Breanna get fat on purpose just so I could put her on a diet and get on TV. *What?*

We read other comments criticizing us for letting this happen and not preventing it before it got this far, and those things were true but hurtful. I had beaten myself up about that plenty already and didn't need anyone else to do it for me.

Other people suspected that I must have put Breanna on a liquid diet or forced her to lose weight in another unhealthy way. It took me weeks to pull myself back together after everything I read.

Here's what I learned from that experience: if you're ever going to put yourself into the public spotlight, don't ever, *ever* read the comments.

· · ·

Breanna's next visit to the doctor was awkward. We'd just shared our journey on national television, and on it, I'd said that our pediatrician had told me that Breanna would grow into her body. In his office now, I wondered if he'd seen the interview.

But he went through the exam as usual. Only at the very end did he say, "By the way, I saw you on TV."

"Oh yeah?" I offered a shaky smile.

He nodded. He didn't say anything else.

After that, it was just too uncomfortable to go back. I found a new pediatrician and explained what we'd been through with our old pediatrician. She was completely dumbfounded by the medical advice we'd received up to this point, particularly when I mentioned the "stunted growth" comment.

"That's actually backward," she said. "Her growth would have been stunted if she *hadn't* lost the weight." She went on to explain that bone and joint damage can occur from carrying around too much extra weight. She also said that she had those tough conversations with patients' parents on a regular basis. It can't be easy to tell a parent, "Your child needs to lose weight," but she did it. I knew then that we were in the right place.

But I can't get lost in those regrets. My focus has to stay on the present and how well Breanna is doing now.

• • •

Breanna's next invitation was to be on *The Biggest Loser* to tell her story as part of their "Challenge America" campaign. The season that we were on the show, they were focusing on bringing awareness to childhood obesity. Even though I was pretty stung by the side effects of having gone public, we all felt it was important to keep sharing our story, knowing that it could help other kids and families who were going through the same thing. We said yes.

We had never seen the show before, but we began watching

it immediately. Right away Breanna related to a woman on the show named Danni Allen. At the beginning of the show, Danni was twenty-six years old and weighed 258 pounds. She'd had weight problems as a kid and had a wake-up call when her father wound up in the hospital and almost died as a result of weight-related problems. She decided that she'd better get serious about losing weight if she didn't want to be at death's door by age fifty.

But she didn't count on how hard it would be to get moving. In the second episode, Jillian Michaels literally dumped a bucket of ice water on her head to get Danni to "wake up."

I liked Jillian's style!

I think Breanna saw a lot of her own journey in Danni's. Not only did they both have so much to lose, but they went through a lot of the same physical challenges too. At first neither one of them wanted to put in the hard work it took to get results. Yet from week to week, I could see the changes in Danni, just as I'd seen the changes in Breanna. It wasn't just her body either—there was a change in her attitude and her demeanor. We felt like we were watching her blossom.

Our whole family rooted for her, and from the start, Breanna declared, "I just know she's going to win."

Make Way for Veggies
Eating fresh produce means lots of trips to the grocery store or farmer's market—probably two or three times a week (unless you choose to stock up on frozen produce). You might want to have a chopping day as a family, where each person takes a cutting board and goes to town on some vegetables. After you're done chopping, you can pack the veggies in Tupperware containers for easy-to-grab snacks or additions to meals. Doing this kind of prep work ahead of time means that making meals won't feel like as much of a chore, and besides, your kids just might think it's fun.

A camera crew had followed us around for a day to film Breanna for an upcoming episode. That season, the show's pediatrician said something that struck me: "The home must be a safe place. [Kids] will have every opportunity to eat junk food outside the home." Truer words have never been said.

As the physician explained, the high-fat, high-salt, high-sugar foods that are so intertwined with childhood are addicting, and they can create a vicious cycle of craving and overeating, undermining any efforts made to solve a weight problem. When Breanna was obese, she wouldn't eat a vegetable because, according to the way her brain was wired, it was competing with the hyperpalatability of the scientifically manufactured foods. A fatty, salty chip is far more rewarding to the brain than raw snap peas—we associate those instant-reward qualities with pleasure. It required a slow detox, but as she consumed less fake food and more real food, she discovered that she actually *liked* real food. She just needed to get used to it.

We were invited to the season finale of *The Biggest Loser*. We immediately recognized faces from the show, and people also recognized Breanna and praised her for her hard work. They treated her like a rock star, and she enjoyed the attention.

Unbeknownst to me, Breanna was on a mission—the kind of mission only a ten-year-old would dare to undertake. She had bought a little trophy from the hotel's gift shop that said, "You're a Super Star" and had carried it with her into the finale. I had no idea what she was planning to do with it. At one point she misplaced it, and I didn't understand why she was so frantic to find it.

We watched the finalists do their last weigh-ins to determine who would be the season 14 winner. It was a nail-biting ending in which the winner was separated from the runner-up by just one pound. Danni won! If you've never seen a *Biggest Loser* finale, it's quite a spectacle. Confetti and streamers descend on the winner, and the press swarms the stage.

Somehow Breanna managed to wiggle her way through the masses of people and ultimately reach Danni.

Breanna called out to her from beside the stage: "Excuse me! Excuse me!"

Danni bent down to Breanna, who produced the little trophy as if it were made of gold.

She handed it to Danni and said, "I want you to have this. I knew you were going to win."

Even from where I stood, I could see the tears in Danni's eyes. "Thank you," she said.

It was quite a moment for Breanna. Here was a woman who had suffered from a profound lack of belief in herself but now stood on that stage as a winner. Breanna understood what it took for Danni to win, because she'd lived a similar journey. It was a precious moment to watch.

When all this media came into our lives, we still weren't done with the weight-loss journey. At the time of the *Good Morning America* show, Bre had lost sixty-six pounds and was down to 120. She hit her goal weight in January 2012: 115 pounds. It had been just over a year since the beginning of our journey. And then . . . she decided to keep going.

CONTESTS AND ACCOUNTABILITY

One of the reasons *The Biggest Loser* is effective is because it provides competition and accountability. Participants have to weigh in every week, and if they don't achieve their goals, their team can suffer and they can lose the chance to win a lot of money.

You might be able to do something similar for your own child. Turning weight loss into a competition can be fun and motivating, as long as it's done in good spirit and with reasonable expectations. In addition to rewards for weight-loss milestones, consider what else you can do to introduce a sense of fun competition into your routine.

Here are some ideas to get you started:

1. Have your child race you around the track.
2. Have a contest to see who can do the most push-ups or sit-ups.
3. Keep a chart of times and records, and have your child try to accomplish personal bests.
4. Make a food chart and see who can make the healthiest food choices for a week.
5. Invite other kids to join you on your journey (cousins, neighbors, and friends).
6. Host competitions in your yard or at the park. Play games like Red Light, Green Light; Duck, Duck, Goose; Monkey in the Middle; tag; and musical chairs. Have three-legged races, relay races, obstacle course races, and mini Olympics events. You might even want to get a bunch of dollar-store prizes for an afternoon of contests.
7. Find someone your child can check in with (besides you) for accountability. Have your child share milestones with that person.

CHAPTER 12

JUST THE BEGINNING

Now that I had successfully tackled dinner, it was time to take on breakfast. Breakfast really is the most important meal of the day—it provides the energy to get you going and the nutrients to sustain you. When you're eating right, you don't need coffee. A fresh smoothie gives you a natural energy boost without the caffeine.

I wanted Breanna and Nathan to get all the nutrients their bodies needed, so I started making breakfast smoothies, using spinach as a base and adding kale and fruit to taste. I invested in a Vitamix blender, which may have been my best purchase on this journey. We use it every day now, but it wasn't an instant hit.

The first time I made smoothies for my kids, I served them in tiny condiment cups—the kind you'd find at a fast-food restaurant for ketchup. That's all I required them to try. Breanna put up with it, but Nathan hated it with a passion. He procrastinated for as long as possible, and I sat with him at the table for an hour waiting for him to drink it. He would insist on plugging his nose with a clip and immediately chasing it down with a glass of water. A few years ago, I surely would have given up. I never would have forced my kids to finish something they didn't like. But now I knew better—not only was it good for them, but they might end up liking it eventually. I was a case in point. Sometimes I still find it hard to believe that I enjoy drinking spinach and kale smoothies for breakfast.

The kids started drinking half a glass of smoothie every morning along with whatever else they were eating, such as steel-cut oatmeal, toast with peanut butter or fresh fruit, or healthier cereal. I drank a full glass. To this day, Nathan doesn't jump with joy over drinking it, but I don't have to talk him into it, either. It's part of our everyday routine, and he knows it will give him a great kick start for his day.

At Breanna's birthday party that year, she celebrated ten years—the big double digits. She'd hit her goal weight a few days prior, and she looked healthy and fit. I couldn't help but think that just fourteen months before, we'd been in a much different place. If someone had told me back then that Breanna wouldn't be overweight anymore, I would have thought they had the wrong person.

For her party food, we put out fruit and veggie platters instead of chips. Breanna made the fruit platter herself. I had a moment of hesitation as I argued with myself about whether or not cake was okay.

It's once a year, and it's her birthday, I said to myself. *Once a year has to be okay, even for Military Mom.*

So we had the cake. One slice each, and then we gave away the leftovers so they wouldn't be sitting around the house tempting us.

• • •

As each season ended, Breanna kept joining additional sports. Her latest was water polo. To my amazement, she now *asked* to join these teams. It was hard to believe this was the same kid who once refused to move. Now she couldn't get enough of it!

What amazes me most is how quickly all this happened. Although it felt like an agonizing process at the time, she'd gone from sedentary to truly athletic in a single year. If I hadn't let her get so heavy in the first place, the process might have gone even faster. That's what was standing between her and her real destiny: one year of exercise and healthy eating.

On March 26, Breanna hit her final goal weight: 110 pounds. She had lost 40 percent of her original body weight. And then, metaphorically speaking, we threw away the scale.

It's important to weigh in weekly when you're in weight-loss mode. It's motivating and keeps you on track as you see what works, what doesn't, and when you need to increase your efforts. But you don't ever want to get so tied to the numbers on the scale that you lose sight of the bigger picture: a healthy, sustainable lifestyle. Now that she had met her goal, it was time to put an end to the weekly weigh-ins. The scale—and Breanna—had earned a break. We had made it through her weight-loss journey, and now we would enter maintenance mode, where the goal is not to lose any more weight but just to maintain her current weight (making adjustments for growth).

People think that there's a big difference between the two, but there's really not. It just means you can ease up a little. Breanna continued all her sports and worked out in the gym three days a week, but she was allowed to go to more events where I knew there would be bad food. I prayed she would limit herself and make good choices.

That summer we planned her weight-loss party—the one we'd talked about for months, the one that had gotten us through some of the really hard times, the one she'd worked so hard to earn. I knew we would get to this moment, but as we were going through everything, this day was hard to imagine. During our walks and runs, we'd talk about what kind of party we would have—who we'd invite, who would be the DJ, what food we'd serve, and what activities we'd do.

We picked a day in August and invited all our closest friends and family. The day of the party, I went shopping to buy the food. As I was walking down the aisle, I saw the sacks of potatoes. An idea came to me: *It would be great if people could actually see and hold how much extra weight Breanna fought so hard to lose!*

As I started grabbing the eighty pounds of potatoes one sack at a time and loaded them onto the cart, a wave of emotion flooded over me. *I can't believe this is how much extra weight Breanna was carrying with her!* It was just a brief exertion for me, yet she hadn't been able to escape that weight as she went about her daily life. She was only nine . . . how could I have been so blind?

It hit me once again that none of this would have happened

if I'd just fed her healthy foods from the start and made sure she got plenty of exercise. I couldn't stop crying as I loaded all eight sacks of potatoes into my car.

I thought back on all that had changed in the past year—she had no more pain in her legs and feet, no rashes or pressure on her belly, no trouble breathing. She no longer got winded going up the stairs. All of those constraints were gone, allowing her to feel as carefree as a kid should feel.

When I got home, I put those eight sacks of potatoes (minus a few—so the weight would be seventy-nine instead of eighty) on a table for everyone to see, with a sign below that read, "Seventy-nine pounds of potatoes: equivalent to the weight Breanna no longer carries with her every day." Some of the guests tried holding the sacks. Only two men could lift them—and only for a brief amount of time.

As an extra surprise, I bought seventy-nine white and yellow balloons to represent each pound she had fought so hard to lose. We gathered together for a group picture with Breanna holding all the balloons. She felt like she might float off into the air . . . the helium lifted her arms right up!

"Okay, when we get to one, let them go," I said.

We all counted down: "Three, two, one!"

It was quite a sight—I'll never forget seeing seventy-nine balloons floating into the blue sky over Clovis. Seventy-nine balloons gone—just like the weight Breanna no longer carries.

The evening was filled with swimming and music and laughter, and we danced into the night under the stars. It gave us all a chance to reflect on what an amazing journey it had been.

"Was it worth it?" I asked Breanna.

"Yes, but I am never going to do that again!"

I gave her a big hug. Those were my thoughts exactly.

• • •

As Breanna's fifth-grade year drew to a close, Dan and I made an important decision: we wanted Breanna to attend her last year of elementary school with a fresh start. We applied for an inter-district transfer to another local elementary school where the only kids who knew her would be friends from swim club. She had never been "the fat girl" there. She was starting sixth grade, so it would give her one last year before junior high where she could be unattached to labels, away from anyone who had ever bullied or teased her.

There were, however, two factors that made our decision difficult. First, she had just made the cheerleading squad, and there was no guarantee that they'd let her on the team at the new school since tryouts were over. The second drawback was more about nostalgia than anything. It would mean we'd no longer be close to our walking trail—the spot where our journey had started. That trail was the place where I'd first realized that we were meant for something better than what we had—the place where I met the woman I was supposed to be. But we discussed our options and decided that it was more important to get Breanna into a new environment.

We didn't know until right before school started whether we'd been approved for the transfer. At the last minute, we heard back: we'd been approved! Both Breanna and Nathan would go to the other elementary school together.

So that September, with her fresh, new pencils in her brand-new backpack, Breanna walked into her new school with her head held high. And this time, she really *was* the new girl. She was nervous about how she'd fit in, but that didn't stop her from getting involved. She joined the cross-country team and the cheerleading squad, and later in the year she earned a spot on the competition cheer team—a huge accomplishment.

Dan wrote letters to both Breanna and Nathan's teachers on the first day of school.

> *Our kids are new to the school, and we're looking forward to a great year. We have one request. Our family is doing all we can to eat well, and we request that our kids not partake in the food provided for parties—treats, candy, etc. If events are planned, we will provide a snack or treat ourselves to prevent them from feeling left out.*
>
> *Thank you,*
> *Daniel and Heidi Bond*

Both teachers agreed, but Breanna's teacher didn't always follow the request. There were several times when I heard about Breanna getting candy, cupcakes, or pizza in class. So many people are of the "oh, it's just one" mind-set. The problem is that "just once" easily turns into once a week. They don't understand that those small indulgences add up and can derail someone with weight issues, especially when she's just getting past the craving for those kinds of foods.

• • •

When sixth grade hit, Breanna was so busy with sports and swimming that our workouts tapered down to three days a week. After a couple of months, I began to rethink our strategy. If Breanna was going to take ownership of fitness in her life—both now and in the future—then it would have to be something she wanted, something she was in control of. The workouts would have to be something she had accomplished herself, not just something she'd done because her mom was right there working out with her.

That's when I told her she was going to have to start doing the workouts on her own. She was ready to embrace that change. We continued working out together from time to time, but most of the time she exercised on her own.

One day the two of us went out on the old trail together, which we hadn't done in almost three months. We were running together when Breanna sped ahead of me. I couldn't keep up.

It was fantastic.

She looked back at me with a questioning look, as if to say, *Should I keep going or wait for you?*

"Go on!" I called. I was filled with awe and gratitude as I watched my little girl run ahead of me. She had been training with her school's cross-country team, and it was paying off. She made it to the end of the trail and then turned around, passing me going the other way.

I wanted to tell her, "Good job! You're awesome!" But I was so out of breath I couldn't say a word. Instead, I just high-fived her as tears of joy ran down my face.

I wasn't the leader anymore. I didn't have to yell back at her to hurry up or to keep up with me or to get moving. The student had surpassed the teacher.

She excelled in both swimming and cross-country. Breanna's

cross-country coach realized that she was best suited for running longer distances, and she was chosen as one of three athletes to represent her school in a district-wide elementary school championship meet. Ironically, her niche is the 1,500 meter—just shy of one mile. That was the exact distance she'd always dreaded in gym class. Two years earlier, she'd completed the mile in gym class in fourteen minutes, panting and out of breath and mostly walking. Now she could do it in six minutes flat.

• • •

I had hoped that once we were done with the weight-loss journey, we'd never have to look back. I was wrong.

Halfway through sixth grade, I noticed that Breanna had gained some weight back that looked like more than what normal growth would account for. We had her weigh in and discovered she had gained back ten pounds. Between the snacks at school and at friends' houses, she had made some bad choices, and it had an immediate impact. When she saw the number on the scale, she was devastated.

It was hard for both of us to see how easy it was to lose ground on all the hard work. Her body had undergone massive changes, but her genetic wiring hadn't changed; she was still prone to putting on weight easily. Her friends could eat junk food and not have to worry about their weight, but indulgences here and there meant a big gain for her, even with all her activity and otherwise healthy eating.

Over the next few weeks we really watched what we ate and limited social events where we knew there would be bad food, and she lost some of the weight. Meanwhile, I wished

I could banish all the Starbursts and Skittles and soda from the world so they wouldn't tempt her or anyone else again.

I took a small stand at one of Breanna's swim meets. Parents are expected to put in a certain amount of volunteer time for the club, and I was usually part of the hospitality crew, which involved handing out water and healthy snacks to the swimmers, coaches, and officials. I preferred that to working in the snack bar, where I'd have to sell junk to kids. One day, at a summer league meet, there wasn't a hospitality team, and when I saw that one of the parents in charge of the snack bar needed help, I volunteered. As I watched the kids and parents come up and buy junk food, I realized that there wasn't even one healthy option they could choose. I asked the man in charge if we could start offering some healthy choices at the snack bar.

"This is what kids want, and it's what makes the club money," he said. "We have to sell what they want."

"Well, how about if I bring in some air-popped popcorn next time and see if that sells too?"

"I wouldn't bother. They're not going to choose that over candy."

He hadn't directly said no, so I decided to give it a shot. I made a big batch of air-popped popcorn, filled about forty-five Ziploc bags, and waited to see what would happen. He was right: most kids chose the unhealthy stuff. But not everybody did—my popcorn sold out.

What I've learned along the way is that some kids and parents will make the right choices when they're given the option. I hope that my kids always will. We've learned what fuels us instead of what robs us of our health, and now we know what's at stake.

For us, maintenance mode is real work. We've been in maintenance mode for a year and a half. One of the best evidences of growth is that Breanna now cares when she has gone off track, which means that I don't have to push so hard. We may never get to a place of coasting, and we may have to consciously choose the path of health day after day. But that will be enough to live the abundant life—and to conquer obesity.

BABY STEPS

It's not realistic to change all your eating habits at once. The more sustainable way is to make small changes in your diet and lifestyle and then keep adding to these changes over time. You might want to start by examining your family's worst eating habits and then replacing them one at a time. If you're not sure where to start, here are some suggestions:

- **Substitute extra-virgin olive oil.** Regardless of what the recipe calls for, extra-virgin olive oil can be substituted for the butter or oil. Substitute the extra-virgin olive oil for about three-fourths the amount of butter listed. So if a recipe calls for one stick of butter (eight tablespoons), use six tablespoons of extra-virgin olive oil. When cooking on the stovetop, use little to no oil. If you must use something, put a couple of drops of extra-virgin olive oil in the pan, and then use a paper towel to spread them around. You might try grilling to avoid using oil, or you might replace oil with a little chicken broth.
- **Never drink your calories.** Your best choices are water or tea.
- **Measure your serving sizes.** A serving of meat should be the size of the palm of your hand (a child's serving should be the size of the palm of his or her own hand).

- **Buy fruits and vegetables that are in season.** They are cheaper and more flavorful, with higher nutritional value. Try to find local farmer's markets if you can. Most produce loses nutrients the longer it sits around, so eat it as fresh as possible. You can also choose frozen fruits and vegetables in the off-season.
- **Add vegetables to everything.** Vegetables are filling, add valuable nutrition, and provide great flavor. If you're not used to eating vegetables at breakfast, try it—you just might be surprised to find you like it! Put peppers or asparagus in omelets, and drink vegetable-based smoothies.
- **Never skip a meal.** It throws off your metabolism, brings down your energy, and makes you more prone to binge eat later.
- **No grazing.** Don't leave food lying around. You don't need a candy dish or a bunch of chips in the pantry. Mealtime is mealtime; watching television isn't time for a bonus meal.
- **Read labels carefully.** The fewer ingredients, the better. Ingredients are listed in the order of quantity, from greatest to least. Sugar should not be one of the first five ingredients.
- **Substitute Greek yogurt.** Greek yogurt has about half the sugar of its traditional counterpart. Nonfat Greek yogurt can often stand in for sour cream, mayonnaise, and heavy cream in recipes. Experiment with your recipes, and you'll be surprised how yummy this alternative can be.
- **Substitute applesauce.** Unsweetened applesauce (or homemade applesauce—see recipe in appendix 2) can stand in for sugar in many recipes, such as banana bread and zucchini bread.

- **Switch to powdered peanut butter.** Regular peanut butter is full of fat and oil. With the powdered stuff, the fat calories are reduced by 85 percent! Even so, don't go crazy with serving sizes. Spread just a thin layer on for a source of protein.
- **Add cinnamon.** Cinnamon adds great flavor and nutritional value; try it sprinkled on applesauce, soup, or a light layer of peanut butter.
- **Throw out your salt shaker.** It will take time, but your taste buds will adjust, and soon you'll be appreciating the flavors that are already in your food.
- **Use fresh herbs.** Fresh herbs make a huge difference in creating flavorful meals. To preserve the leftovers, place the herbs in an ice cube tray with a small amount of extra-virgin olive oil. When frozen, transfer them to a plastic bag and keep in the freezer for future use. You can toss one right into the pan when you cook your meals.
- **Keep a cutting board on display.** Have it out and handy so you remember to use it frequently to cut up fresh fruits and veggies.
- **Always have dried mint on hand.** It's great for digestion and adds wonderful flavor to tea.
- **Puree spinach and freeze it in an ice cube tray.** This makes for an easy add-in for soups, side dishes, and more.
- **Drink a glass of water before every meal** and stay hydrated throughout the day.
- **Never bring leftovers home.** It's fine to indulge at a restaurant every now and then, but you don't need to indulge the next day, too.
- **Use nutritional yeast** if you want to add a little flavor to air-popped popcorn.

- **Shop the perimeter.** When shopping, try not to venture
  into the middle of the store. Keep your purchases to
  the perimeter—fresh fruits, fresh vegetables, meats,
  and a limited amount of dairy products. The junk (chips,
  cookies, processed foods) is in the middle!
- **Plan ahead.** Think through your day and have your food
  packed and ready before you leave the house. Never go
  to a water park or entertainment venue without healthy
  snacks.
- **Live life.** Once in maintenance mode, live life. If your
  child is invited to a birthday party, discuss in advance
  what and how much he or she will eat. Life happens, and
  food is often a part of socializing. Kids need to learn to
  make smart choices at social events.

YES, YOU CAN!

MY DAUGHTER JUST QUALIFIED for the Junior Olympics in swimming.

It's hard to believe this is the same girl who rarely got up off the couch and struggled to climb the stairs. When I stop and think back over our journey, it feels like a miracle.

While I used to be the one pushing Breanna, she is now the one pushing herself to try new things and see what she can achieve. The summer after fifth grade, she completed her first junior triathlon—a 150-meter swim followed by a four-mile bike ride and then a one-mile run. By the time she neared the finish line, she was so exhausted she thought she would collapse, but she made it. She finished in third place for her age group and got to stand on the winners' podium.

I had no idea there was a hidden athlete in my daughter, buried so deeply in her too-big body. She had no idea, either.

Breanna and I recently went camping by ourselves, back to the Happy Isles trail at Yosemite.

This time, when we got to the end of the trail, she looked at me with raised eyebrows. "That's it?" she said. "That was the whole trail?"

"It feels different, doesn't it?"

"No kidding."

We decided to keep going. This time we went to the top of Vernal Fall to see the waterfall from above. It was an incredible view that we never would have seen before this weight-loss journey. And that's what it's been about all along—learning to see life from a new angle and loving the view.

For so many years, obesity was like a cancer that had taken control of us. Now it's not even part of our lives. With that burden lifted, I am finally free to let go of most of my worries. I will always have some level of concern about what happens to Breanna when she goes off to college and then out on her own—will she continue to make the right choices if I'm not there to stand over her and enforce consequences?

But I trust that she cares about her health now and doesn't ever want to go back to where she was before. I have to believe that if she falters, it won't be a significant fall, and that she'll know how to get back on track again.

• • •

One day, after we'd been in maintenance mode for a while, I woke up with this rather startling realization: *If I don't have to spend my time worrying about obesity, what will I do with my life?*

I had been so focused on my mission, and for a long time that goal line seemed light-years away. One hundred and ten pounds? I believed we'd get there, but it was a nebulous, faraway ideal—until suddenly it was reality. I was no longer sure what to do with myself. I thanked God for giving us the strength to complete the journey, because there were times of doubt and times when it took more strength than I thought I had. And then I sensed him telling me that it was time to enjoy the fruits of our labors.

Now I could go to Breanna's and Nathan's sporting events just like any other mom—not with bated breath, hoping this would work, but with the joy of watching my kids compete and have fun. And my own fitness was no longer just about leading my daughter; it was about keeping healthy for my own sake. And I could start following the dreams I didn't even know I had.

I started to realize that if we could do something that formerly seemed impossible, then there must be other "impossibles" out there for me to break down. One of my biggest hopes now is to open a weight-loss center for kids, teens, and parents. It would include an indoor track for walking, jogging, and running; a trampoline arena; treadmills; a dodgeball court; and an Olympic-size pool. The gym was an integral part of our journey, but I wish we'd had access to a place without age restrictions, built with kids in mind. Considering that childhood obesity is now an epidemic in the United States, I know there are countless

Not Sure Where to Start? We love swimming because it's a full-body workout, and it's not hard on joints and bones, with a low risk of injury. Try www.swimtoday.org to find a club near your home.

other families like ours who would benefit from a resource like this.

It's a big goal, but if you're going to dream, dream big! After all, Disneyland wasn't built in a day.

So we've started taking baby steps in that direction. Breanna is mentoring kids who want help losing weight, and I've opened up our home gym to anyone who wants to use it. I'm starting to do some public speaking about how to fight childhood obesity, and this book is another step on that journey. It's so important to both Breanna and me that we use our experience to help others. No one should go through something like this feeling as helpless and alone as we did in the beginning.

• • •

Getting to this point required a complete attitude change for all of us. We went through the first nine years of Breanna's life thinking, *We can't* and the past three years knowing, *We can*. It's dangerous to pigeonhole ourselves or our kids—to start assuming we're lazy, unathletic, or hopeless. Each person has so much untapped potential inside. The question is, will we choose to call that out in ourselves and in the people we love?

The victories that mean the most are those that are hard won. Through faith and determination, we conquered the demon that held our family hostage for so long, and I got my daughter back. It taught me that when you keep putting one foot in front of the other toward your goal, *anything* is possible.

What I wish for more than anything now is to spread a message of hope to parents and other concerned adults who are experiencing what we went through. Obesity is 100 percent treatable, fixable, and curable. It takes dedication and hard work, but it is *not* a life sentence! My daughter is living proof that with a pair of tennis shoes and some motivation, you can choose a brand-new life.

FORTY-DAY MEAL AND EXERCISE PLAN

BEFORE YOU BEGIN

It can feel overwhelming to change your family's diet. One of the best ways you can get started is to write down everything—yes, *everything*—your child eats. Try doing this for a couple of days before you begin implementing changes so you can get an idea of what normal is now. For each food—including even a little a bite of this or that and all snacks and drinks—record the fat and sugar content. You can also note the calories, but it's not necessary.

Keeping a food journal may sound daunting, but it's not hard to find this kind of information. There are several places online that provide comprehensive databases of just about any food that's commercially available. We like www.fatsecret.com and www.calorieking.com. To find out information about a certain food, just type the food into the search box. You can use specific brand names (for example, "Campbell's creamy tomato soup"), or you can be more generic ("oatmeal"). Then you click on the listing to find the nutrition facts label—the calories, fat content, sugar, sodium, protein, and more.

Even when you know there's a problem, it's eye opening to see everything in black and white and realize just how much your children may be overeating.

For the next two days, write down everything your child eats, without trying to fix it at this point. Once you start seeing problem areas, you can begin making changes and launch the forty-day meal and exercise plan. You can keep track of your notes here, in a notebook, or online. Here are some of the most popular online food diaries: www.fitday.com, www.myfooddiary.com, and www.livestrong.com/myplate.

These sites provide a place to track your food intake and exercise, and some also offer goal-setting tools, a weight tracker, exercise videos, and motivational tips. Whatever system you choose, write it down. Recording everything can help you catch problem spots and figure out where you need to improve.

Day 1

Date: ....

Breakfast: ....

Lunch: ....

Snacks: ....

Dinner: ....

Beverages: ....

Other: ....

Total fat: ....

Total sugar: ....

Day 2

Date: ....

Breakfast: ....

Lunch: ....

Snacks: ....

Dinner: ....

Beverages: ....

Other: ....

Total fat: ....

Total sugar: ....

INITIAL WEIGH-IN:

LET'S GET STARTED!

There is no one right plan when it comes to food and exercise—you'll experiment and find out what works best for you and your family as you go. The important thing is to start making healthy choices and then stay committed to them. My goal is to share what worked for us and give you some different options to try.

This forty-day plan includes suggested exercises and ideas for healthy meals and snacks for each day. You may need to adapt them to fit your family's needs, but hopefully this will get you going in the right direction.

Note that the recipes for the meal suggestions can be found in appendix 2 (page 257), and a shopping list can be found in appendix 3 (page 291).

DAY 1

SUGGESTED MEAL PLAN

Breakfast
low-sugar granola or whole-grain cereal
small Green Smoothie (recipe on p. 258)

Lunch
Bruschetta (recipe on p. 266)

Snack
1 small apple

Dinner
grilled fish
brown rice
veggies

EXERCISE
Walk for 60 minutes (outside or on a treadmill).
Participate in an organized sport, such as swimming or
basketball.

Food Journal

Breakfast: ....

Lunch: ....

Snacks: ....

Dinner: ....

Beverages: ....

Other: ....

Total fat: ....

Total sugar: ....

God is faithful; he will not let you be tempted beyond
what you can bear.   I CORINTHIANS 10:13

DAY 2

SUGGESTED MEAL PLAN

Breakfast

Veggie Omelet (recipe on p. 259)

Lunch

Ham and Swiss Wrap (recipe on p. 270)
carrots with hummus

Snack

pineapple slices

Dinner

Grilled Chicken and Veggie Skewers (recipe on p. 273)
brown rice

EXERCISE

Get an exercise video online or from the library and work out
for 60 minutes.

Food Journal

Breakfast: ....

Lunch: ....

Snacks: ....

Dinner: ....

Beverages: ....

Other: ....

Total fat: ....

Total sugar: ....

*He who began a good work in you will carry it on
to completion until the day of Christ Jesus.*

PHILIPPIANS 1:6

DAY 3

SUGGESTED MEAL PLAN

Breakfast

toast with peanut butter, cinnamon, and raspberries

Lunch

Potato Kale Soup (recipe on p. 284)

Snack

sliced strawberries

Dinner

Ranch Chicken with Corn on the Cob (recipe on p. 276)
baked potato
side salad

EXERCISE

Walk for 60 minutes.
Participate in an organized sport.

Food Journal

Breakfast: ....

Lunch: ....

Snacks: ....

Dinner: ....

Beverages: ....

Other: ....

Total fat: ....

Total sugar: ....

*I have learned the secret of being content in any and
every situation, whether well fed or hungry.*

PHILIPPIANS 4:12

DAY 4

SUGGESTED MEAL PLAN

Breakfast

small Green Smoothie
yogurt
fruit

Lunch

shaved chicken sandwich
celery sticks with ranch

Snack

1 banana

Dinner

ground beef tacos
sliced strawberries

EXERCISE

Ride your bike for 60 minutes or do a 60-minute circuit workout in your house (alternate between stair-climbing, jumping jacks, push-ups, and sit-ups).
Participate in an organized sport.

Food Journal

Breakfast: ....

Lunch: ....

Snacks: ....

Dinner: ....

Beverages: ....

Other: ....

Total fat: ....

Total sugar: ....

See to it that no one takes you captive through hollow and deceptive philosophy.   COLOSSIANS 2:8

DAY 5

SUGGESTED MEAL PLAN

Breakfast

egg
toast with fruit spread

Lunch

pastrami wrap
celery sticks with hummus

Snack

1 small serving of grapes

Dinner

shrimp nachos loaded with veggies

EXERCISE

Walk for 60 minutes.

Participate in an organized sport.

Food Journal

    Breakfast: ....

    Lunch: ....

    Snacks: ....

    Dinner: ....

    Beverages: ....

    Other: ....

    Total fat: ....

    Total sugar: ....

Set your minds on things above, not on earthly things.

COLOSSIANS 3:2

DAY 6

SUGGESTED MEAL PLAN

Breakfast

½ papaya squirted with lime juice

cottage cheese

Lunch

grilled chicken

side salad

Snack

1 peach

Dinner

Breanna's Cheeseburgers (recipe on p. 279)
pickle wedges

EXERCISE

Walk for 60 minutes.
Get an exercise video online or from the library and work out
for 60 minutes.

Food Journal

Breakfast: ....

Lunch: ....

Snacks: ....

Dinner: ....

Beverages: ....

Other: ....

Total fat: ....

Total sugar: ....

Rejoice always, pray continually, give thanks in all circumstances; for this is God's will for you in Christ Jesus. I THESSALONIANS 5:16-18

DAY 7

SUGGESTED MEAL PLAN

Breakfast
small Green Smoothie
1 slice of toast with peanut butter and sliced peaches (broiled, if you like)

Lunch
grilled cheese
carrots

Snack
air-popped popcorn

Dinner
Grilled Asian Steak (recipe on p. 278)
salad
Healthy Cauliflower "Mashed Potatoes" (recipe on p. 287)

ACTIVITY
Go roller-skating or ice-skating as a family.

Food Journal

Breakfast: ....

Lunch: ....

Snacks: ....

Dinner: ....

Beverages: ....

Other: ....

Total fat: ....

Total sugar: ....

Faith is confidence in what we hope for and assurance about what we do not see.

HEBREWS 11:1

WEEK 1 WEIGH-IN:

DAY 8

SUGGESTED MEAL PLAN

Breakfast

oatmeal with fruit and honey

Lunch

Chicken Quesadilla (recipe on p. 263)

Snack

rice cake

Dinner

chicken tacos loaded with veggies

EXERCISE

Walk for 60 minutes. This week, work toward four miles per hour in your walking. Use your arms to speed-walk as much as possible or set the treadmill to four miles per hour.
Participate in an organized sport.

Food Journal

Breakfast: ....

Lunch: ....

Snacks: ....

Dinner: ....

Beverages: ....

Other: ....

Total fat: ....

Total sugar: ....

No discipline seems pleasant at the time, but painful.
Later on, however, it produces a harvest of righteousness
and peace. HEBREWS 12:11

DAY 9

SUGGESTED MEAL PLAN

Breakfast

small Green Smoothie
whole-grain cereal

Lunch

sandwich with peanut butter and fruit spread
orange slices

Snack

1 small apple

Dinner

Make-Your-Own Pizza (recipe on p. 270)
salad

EXERCISE

Get an exercise video online or from the library and work out
for 60 minutes.
Participate in an organized sport.

Food Journal

Breakfast: ....

Lunch: ....

Snacks: ....

Dinner: ....

Beverages: ....

Other: ....

Total fat: ....

Total sugar: ....

*Consider it pure joy, my brothers and sisters, whenever
you face trials of many kinds, because you know that the
testing of your faith produces perseverance.*

JAMES 1:2-3

DAY 10

SUGGESTED MEAL PLAN

Breakfast

cottage cheese
fresh peach slices with cinnamon

Lunch

Cheesy Barbecue Chicken Tortillas (recipe on p. 279)

Snack

carrots with hummus

Dinner

shrimp skewers
brown rice
side salad

EXERCISE

Walk for 60 minutes.
Participate in an organized sport.

Food Journal

Breakfast: ....

Lunch: ....

Snacks: ....

Dinner: ....

Beverages: ....

Other: ....

Total fat: ....

Total sugar: ....

This is the confidence we have in approaching God: that if we ask anything according to his will, he hears us. I JOHN 5:14

DAY 11

SUGGESTED MEAL PLAN

Breakfast

one small pancake with sliced strawberries and Strawberry Sauce (recipe on p. 260)
small Green Smoothie

Lunch

Ranch Chicken
fruit
raw carrots with low-fat ranch dressing

Snack

1 peach

Dinner

ground beef tacos loaded with veggies

EXERCISE

Ride your bike for 60 minutes or do a 60-minute circuit workout
in your house (alternate between stair-climbing, jumping jacks,
push-ups, and sit-ups).
Participate in an organized sport.

Food Journal

Breakfast: ....

Lunch: ....

Snacks: ....

Dinner: ....

Beverages: ....

Other: ....

Total fat: ....

Total sugar: ....

*The LORD himself goes before you and will be with you;
he will never leave you nor forsake you.*

DEUTERONOMY 31:8

DAY 12

SUGGESTED MEAL PLAN

Breakfast

low-sugar granola or whole-grain cereal
small Green Smoothie

Lunch

Chicken Nachos (recipe on p. 283)

Snack

1 nectarine

Dinner

baked turkey breast
Healthy Cauliflower "Mashed Potatoes" with a little grated
Parmesan on top
green beans

EXERCISE

Walk for 60 minutes.
Participate in an organized sport.

Food Journal

Breakfast: ....

Lunch: ....

Snacks: ....

Dinner: ....

Beverages: ....

Other: ....

Total fat: ....

Total sugar: ....

Peace I leave with you; my peace I give you. . . . Do not let your hearts be troubled and do not be afraid.

JOHN 14:27

DAY 13

SUGGESTED MEAL PLAN

Breakfast

Peachy Cinnamon Bread (recipe on p. 261)
yogurt

Lunch

cooked tofu sprinkled with nutritional yeast
side salad

Snack

1 small serving of grapes

Dinner

barbecue chicken
baked potato
salad

EXERCISE

Walk for 60 minutes.

Get an exercise video online or from the library and work out for 60 minutes.

Food Journal

Breakfast: ....

Lunch: ....

Snacks: ....

Dinner: ....

Beverages: ....

Other: ....

Total fat: ....

Total sugar: ....

"I know the plans I have for you," declares the LORD, "plans to prosper you and not to harm you, plans to give you hope and a future."

JEREMIAH 29:11

DAY 14

SUGGESTED MEAL PLAN

Breakfast

Simple Scrambled Egg (recipe on p. 258)
one slice of toast

Lunch

Grilled Honey and Soy Sauce Chicken (recipe on p. 282)
brown rice
veggies

Snack

air-popped popcorn

Dinner

shrimp and veggie skewers

ACTIVITY

Walk to the park as a family and throw a Frisbee or play a game of tag. If the weather doesn't cooperate, play Wii Fit together or go swimming at an indoor pool.

Food Journal

Breakfast: ....

Lunch: ....

Snacks: ....

Dinner: ....

Beverages: ....

Other: ....

Total fat: ....

Total sugar: ....

[Jesus said,] "I have told you these things, so that in me you may have peace." JOHN 16:33

WEEK 2 WEIGH-IN:

DAY 15

SUGGESTED MEAL PLAN

Breakfast

oatmeal with fresh strawberries and honey

Lunch

Asian Chicken Pita (recipe on p. 267)
carrots

Snack

sliced apple

Dinner

Grilled Asian Steak
Healthy Fried Rice (recipe on p. 271)
sliced oranges

EXERCISE

Walk for 60 minutes. This week, begin adding jogging to your walks. To start, jog for thirty seconds every five minutes, or use a measuring stick like we did ("Three trees!"). Over the course of an hour, this means twelve brief jogging sessions.
Participate in an organized sport.

Food Journal

Breakfast: ....

Lunch: ....

Snacks: ....

Dinner: ....

Beverages: ....

Other: ....

Total fat: ....

Total sugar: ....

Great peace have those who love your law, and nothing can make them stumble.   PSALM 119:165

DAY 16

SUGGESTED MEAL PLAN

Breakfast

tortilla wrap with 1 egg, cheese, and salsa

Lunch

ham and cheese wrap
celery sticks

Snack

Pineapple Delight (recipe on p. 290)

Dinner

Meat Loaf (recipe on p. 274)
Healthy Cauliflower "Mashed Potatoes"
Parmesan Spinach (recipe on p. 286)

EXERCISE

Walk for 60 minutes or work out with an exercise video for 60 minutes.
Participate in an organized sport.

Food Journal

Breakfast: ....

Lunch: ....

Snacks: ....

Dinner: ....

Beverages: ....

Other: ....

Total fat: ....

Total sugar: ....

Do not fear, for I am with you; do not be dismayed, for I am your God. ISAIAH 41:10

DAY 17

SUGGESTED MEAL PLAN

Breakfast
oatmeal with blueberries and honey

Lunch
turkey sandwich
carrots with ranch

Snack
1 banana

Dinner
barbecue chicken
veggie skewers
brown rice

EXERCISE
Walk for 60 minutes.
Participate in an organized sport.

Food Journal

Breakfast: ....

Lunch: ....

Snacks: ....

Dinner: ....

Beverages: ....

Other: ....

Total fat: ....

Total sugar: ....

The LORD gives strength to his people; the LORD blesses his people with peace. PSALM 29:11

DAY 18

SUGGESTED MEAL PLAN

Breakfast

small Green Smoothie
toast with peanut butter, banana, and cinnamon

Lunch

grilled cheese
fruit

Snack

1 small apple

Dinner

brown rice pasta with marinara and mushroom sauce
side salad

EXERCISE

Ride your bike for 60 minutes or do a 60-minute circuit workout in your house (alternate between stair-climbing, jumping jacks, push-ups, and sit-ups).

Participate in an organized sport.

Food Journal

Breakfast: ....

Lunch: ....

Snacks: ....

Dinner: ....

Beverages: ....

Other: ....

Total fat: ....

Total sugar: ....

The Spirit God gave us does not make us timid, but gives us power, love and self-discipline.

2 TIMOTHY 1:7

DAY 19

SUGGESTED MEAL PLAN

Breakfast

whole-grain English muffin with 1 egg and a little cheese sprinkled on top

blackberries

Lunch

½ ham sandwich
veggie soup

Snack

carrots with hummus

Dinner

Chicken and Mushrooms (recipe on p. 277)

EXERCISE

Walk for 60 minutes.
Participate in an organized sport.

Food Journal

Breakfast: ....

Lunch: ....

Snacks: ....

Dinner: ....

Beverages: ....

Other: ....

Total fat: ....

Total sugar: ....

*Taste and see that the LORD is good; blessed is the one
who takes refuge in him.* PSALM 34:8

DAY 20

SUGGESTED MEAL PLAN

Breakfast

low-sugar granola or whole-grain cereal
small Green Smoothie

Lunch

Bruschetta

Snack

rice cake

Dinner

Breanna's Cheeseburgers
apple

EXERCISE

Walk for 60 minutes.
Get an exercise video online or from the library and work out
for 60 minutes.

Food Journal

Breakfast: ....

Lunch: ....

Snacks: ....

Dinner: ....

Beverages: ....

Other: ....

Total fat: ....

Total sugar: ....

Trust in the LORD with all your heart, and lean not on your own understanding; in all your ways acknowledge Him, and He shall direct your paths.

PROVERBS 3:5-6, NKJV

DAY 21

SUGGESTED MEAL PLAN

Breakfast

French toast strips topped with berries and strawberry sauce

Lunch

Make-Your-Own Pizza

Snack

Blueberry "Ice Cream" (recipe on p. 289)

Dinner

Teriyaki Chicken (recipe on p. 275)
brown rice
squash

ACTIVITY

If the weather is warm, go to a nearby lake or river and hike. If the weather is cold, bundle up and take a walk or go cross-country skiing.

Food Journal

Breakfast: ....

Lunch: ....

Snacks: ....

Dinner: ....

Beverages: ....

Other: ....

Total fat: ....

Total sugar: ....

If God is for us, who can be against us?
ROMANS 8:31

WEEK 3 WEIGH-IN:

DAY 22

SUGGESTED MEAL PLAN

Breakfast

eggs with cheese and salsa
toast

Lunch

Cheesy Barbecue Chicken Tortillas

Snack

applesauce

Dinner

Grilled Chicken and Veggie Skewers

EXERCISE

Walk for 60 minutes. As you are able, make the jogging bursts longer.
Participate in an organized sport.

Food Journal

Breakfast: ....

Lunch: ....

Snacks: ....

Dinner: ....

Beverages: ....

Other: ....

Total fat: ....

Total sugar: ....

When I cried out for help, you answered me. You made me bold and energized me. PSALM 138:3, NET

DAY 23

SUGGESTED MEAL PLAN

Breakfast
oatmeal with blueberries and honey
small Green Smoothie

Lunch
grilled cheese and ham
carrots

Snack
sliced pineapple

Dinner
Grilled Asian Steak
brown rice
spinach

EXERCISE
Walk for 60 minutes or work out with an exercise video for
60 minutes.
Participate in an organized sport.

Food Journal

Breakfast: ....

Lunch: ....

Snacks: ....

Dinner: ....

Beverages: ....

Other: ....

Total fat: ....

Total sugar: ....

Jesus . . . said, "With man this is impossible, but with God all things are possible." MATTHEW 19:26

DAY 24

SUGGESTED MEAL PLAN

Breakfast

toast with peanut butter and fruit spread

Lunch

Asian Chicken Salad (recipe on p. 272)

Snack

air-popped popcorn

Dinner

Make-Your-Own Pizza loaded with veggies

EXERCISE

Walk for 60 minutes.

Participate in an organized sport.

Food Journal

Breakfast: ....

Lunch: ....

Snacks: ....

Dinner: ....

Beverages: ....

Other: ....

Total fat: ....

Total sugar: ....

Even if our physical body is wearing away, our inner person is being renewed day by day.

2 CORINTHIANS 4:16, NET

DAY 25

SUGGESTED MEAL PLAN

Breakfast

1 egg
cottage cheese with sliced peaches

Lunch

grilled cheese
veggie soup

Snack

berries

Dinner

Pot Roast in Mushroom Sauce (recipe on p. 276)
side salad

EXERCISE

Ride your bike for 60 minutes or do a 60-minute circuit workout
in your house (alternate between stair-climbing, jumping jacks,
push-ups, and sit-ups).
Participate in an organized sport.

Food Journal

Breakfast: ....

Lunch: ....

Snacks: ....

Dinner: ....

Beverages: ....

Other: ....

Total fat: ....

Total sugar: ....

You came near when I called you, and you said,
"Do not fear." LAMENTATIONS 3:57

DAY 26

SUGGESTED MEAL PLAN

Breakfast

Greek yogurt
fresh fruit
small Green Smoothie

Lunch

Ham and Swiss Wrap
apples

Snack

rice cake

Dinner

Beef Kabobs (recipe on p. 281)
brown rice

EXERCISE

Walk for 60 minutes.
Participate in an organized sport.

Food Journal

Breakfast: ....

Lunch: ....

Snacks: ....

Dinner: ....

Beverages: ....

Other: ....

Total fat: ....

Total sugar: ....

You created my inmost being. . . . I praise you because
I am fearfully and wonderfully made.

PSALM 139:13-14

DAY 27

SUGGESTED MEAL PLAN

Breakfast

whole-grain cereal
small Green Smoothie

Lunch

sandwich with peanut butter, banana, and cinnamon
celery sticks

Snack

snack-sized box of raisins

Dinner

Orange and Honey Baked Chicken (recipe on p. 282)
Baked Cauliflower (recipe on p. 286)
steamed broccoli

EXERCISE

Walk for 60 minutes.

Get an exercise video online or from the library and work out for 60 minutes.

Food Journal

Breakfast: ....

Lunch: ....

Snacks: ....

Dinner: ....

Beverages: ....

Other: ....

Total fat: ....

Total sugar: ....

If we ask anything according to his will, he hears us.
1 JOHN 5:14

DAY 28

SUGGESTED MEAL PLAN

Breakfast

oatmeal with bananas and honey

Lunch

Chef's Salad (recipe on p. 264)

Snack

celery sticks with hummus

Dinner

Grilled Honey and Soy Sauce Chicken
brown rice
salad

ACTIVITY

Play racquetball or tennis as a family.

Food Journal

Breakfast: ....

Lunch: ....

Snacks: ....

Dinner: ....

Beverages: ....

Other: ....

Total fat: ....

Total sugar: ....

*He gives strength to the weary and increases the power
of the weak. . . . They will soar on wings like eagles.*

ISAIAH 40:29, 31

WEEK 4 WEIGH-IN:

DAY 29

SUGGESTED MEAL PLAN

Breakfast

1 piece of turkey bacon
slice of toast with peanut butter and fruit

Lunch

½ turkey sandwich
veggie soup

Snack

air-popped popcorn

Dinner

Chicken Nachos loaded with veggies

EXERCISE

Walk/jog for 60 minutes. Try to increase the jogging bursts to forty-five seconds; keep pushing beyond your comfort zone. Participate in an organized sport.

Food Journal

Breakfast: ....

Lunch: ....

Snacks: ....

Dinner: ....

Beverages: ....

Other: ....

Total fat: ....

Total sugar: ....

He heals the brokenhearted and binds up their wounds.
PSALM 147:3

DAY 30

SUGGESTED MEAL PLAN

Breakfast

whole-grain cereal
sliced strawberries

Lunch

Asian Shrimp Spring Rolls (recipe on p. 268)

Snack

sliced fresh peaches

Dinner

grilled steak
No-Fry French Fries (recipe on p. 287)
side salad

EXERCISE
Walk/jog for 60 minutes or work out with an exercise video for 60 minutes.
Participate in an organized sport.

Food Journal

Breakfast: ....

Lunch: ....

Snacks: ....

Dinner: ....

Beverages: ....

Other: ....

Total fat: ....

Total sugar: ....

Be strong and courageous. Do not be afraid or terrified . . . for the LORD your God goes with you.

DEUTERONOMY 31:6

DAY 31

SUGGESTED MEAL PLAN

Breakfast
toast with peanut butter and cinnamon
small Green Smoothie

Lunch

Chef's Salad

Snack

Blueberry "Ice Cream"

Dinner

Orange and Honey Baked Chicken
broccoli
salad

EXERCISE

Walk/jog for 60 minutes.
Participate in an organized sport.

Food Journal

Breakfast: ....

Lunch: ....

Snacks: ....

Dinner: ....

Beverages: ....

Other: ....

Total fat: ....

Total sugar: ....

*I keep my eyes always on the LORD. With him at my
right hand, I will not be shaken.* PSALM 16:8

DAY 32

SUGGESTED MEAL PLAN

Breakfast
oatmeal with banana and honey

Lunch
Ham and Swiss Wrap
carrots with ranch

Snack
1 small apple

Dinner
Pot Roast in Mushroom Sauce
small baked potato
green beans

EXERCISE
Ride your bike for 60 minutes or do a 60-minute circuit workout
in your house (alternate between stair-climbing, jumping jacks,
push-ups, and sit-ups).
Participate in an organized sport.

Food Journal

Breakfast: ....

Lunch: ....

Snacks: ....

Dinner: ....

Beverages: ....

Other: ....

Total fat: ....

Total sugar: ....

Do not be anxious about anything, but in every situation . . . present your requests to God.
PHILIPPIANS 4:6

DAY 33

SUGGESTED MEAL PLAN

Breakfast

1 scrambled egg
cottage cheese
sliced tomatoes

Lunch

steak strips
brown rice
small apple

Snack

rice cake

Dinner

chicken tacos
sliced pineapple

EXERCISE

Ride your bike for 60 minutes or do a 60-minute circuit workout in your house (alternate between stair-climbing, jumping jacks, push-ups, and sit-ups).

Participate in an organized sport.

Food Journal

Breakfast: ....

Lunch: ....

Snacks: ....

Dinner: ....

Beverages: ....

Other: ....

Total fat: ....

Total sugar: ....

Stand firm, and you will win life.
LUKE 21:19

DAY 34

SUGGESTED MEAL PLAN

Breakfast

oatmeal with raspberries and honey

Lunch

sandwich with peanut butter and fresh strawberries

Snack

1 serving of grapes

Dinner

Make-Your-Own Pizza
side salad

EXERCISE

Walk/jog for 60 minutes.
Get an exercise video online or from the library and work out for 60 minutes.

Food Journal

Breakfast: ....

Lunch: ....

Snacks: ....

Dinner: ....

Beverages: ....

Other: ....

Total fat: ....

Total sugar: ....

A wise child accepts a parent's discipline.
PROVERBS 13:1, NLT

DAY 35

SUGGESTED MEAL PLAN

Breakfast

small Green Smoothie
Veggie Omelet

Lunch

Bruschetta

Snack

sliced oranges

Dinner

grilled fish
brown rice
artichokes

ACTIVITY

Go to a playground or an inflatable play center as a family.

Food Journal

Breakfast: ....

Lunch: ....

Snacks: ....

Dinner: ....

Beverages: ....

Other: ....

Total fat: ....

Total sugar: ....

Be joyful in hope, patient in affliction, faithful in prayer. ROMANS 12:12

WEEK 5 WEIGH-IN:

DAY 36

SUGGESTED MEAL PLAN

Breakfast

turkey bacon
toast with peanut butter and blueberries

Lunch

Asian Chicken Pita
sliced strawberries

Snack

kale chips

Dinner

Ranch Chicken with Corn on the Cob
baked potatoes
green beans

EXERCISE

Walk/jog for 60 minutes. Your goal is to gradually work your way up to ten minutes of walking followed by ten minutes of running. Participate in an organized sport.

Food Journal

Breakfast: ....

Lunch: ....

Snacks: ....

Dinner: ....

Beverages: ....

Other: ....

Total fat: ....

Total sugar: ....

Let us not become weary in doing good, for at the proper time we will reap a harvest if we do not give up.
GALATIANS 6:9

DAY 37

SUGGESTED MEAL PLAN

Breakfast

Simple Scrambled Egg
toast

Lunch

grilled ham and cheese
carrots with ranch

Snack

orange slices

Dinner

steak
brown rice
spinach salad

EXERCISE

Walk/jog for 60 minutes or work out with an exercise video for
60 minutes.
Participate in an organized sport.

Food Journal

Breakfast: ....

Lunch: ....

Snacks: ....

Dinner: ....

Beverages: ....

Other: ....

Total fat: ....

Total sugar: ....

Your word is a lamp for my feet, a light on my path.
PSALM 119:105

DAY 38

SUGGESTED MEAL PLAN

Breakfast
tortilla with eggs, spinach, and salsa

Lunch
chicken sandwich
celery sticks with ranch

Snack
sliced strawberries

Dinner
Orange and Honey Baked Chicken
Healthy Fried Rice

EXERCISE
Walk/jog for 60 minutes.
Participate in an organized sport.

Food Journal

Breakfast: ....

Lunch: ....

Snacks: ....

Dinner: ....

Beverages: ....

Other: ....

Total fat: ....

Total sugar: ....

Do not work for food that spoils, but for food that endures to eternal life, which the Son of Man will give you.

JOHN 6:27

DAY 39

SUGGESTED MEAL PLAN

Breakfast

French Toast with blueberries and strawberry sauce (recipe on p. 261)

Lunch

Make-Your-Own Pizza
carrots

Snack

celery with hummus

Dinner

Potato Kale Soup
½ turkey sandwich

EXERCISE

Ride your bike for 60 minutes or do a 60-minute circuit workout in your house (alternate between stair-climbing, jumping jacks, push-ups, and sit-ups).

Participate in an organized sport.

Food Journal

Breakfast: ....

Lunch: ....

Snacks: ....

Dinner: ....

Beverages: ....

Other: ....

Total fat: ....

Total sugar: ....

If you have faith as small as a mustard seed, you can say to this mountain, "Move from here to there," and it will move. Nothing will be impossible for you.

MATTHEW 17:20

DAY 40

SUGGESTED MEAL PLAN

Breakfast

whole-grain cereal

small Green Smoothie

Lunch

Canadian Bacon Quesadilla (recipe on p. 263)
celery sticks with ranch

Snack

applesauce

Dinner

Grilled Honey and Soy Sauce Chicken
Baked Cauliflower
corn

EXERCISE

Walk/jog for 60 minutes.
Participate in an organized sport.

Food Journal

Breakfast:	....
Lunch:	....
Snacks:	....
Dinner:	....
Beverages:	....
Other:	....
Total fat:	....
Total sugar:	....

*Be strong and do not give up, for your work will
be rewarded.* 2 CHRONICLES 15:7

DAY 40 WEIGH-IN:

General Meal-Planning Guidelines

- When the menu refers to toast or sandwiches, use sprouted whole-grain bread.
- When the menu refers to peanut butter, use powdered peanut butter mixed with water, not the high-fat, processed stuff.
- When serving eggs, don't serve more than one full egg (with yolk). If you're making more than one egg, remove the additional yolks because they contain the fat and cholesterol. Another option is to use egg substitute.
- When choosing a salad dressing, make sure it's low fat or fat free, but also make sure it doesn't contain high-fructose corn syrup or a lot of sugar. Manufacturers often add these sweeteners when they take out fat. Look for products that list only natural ingredients on the label.
- Hummus should have 2.5 grams of fat or less per serving.
- You can make your own air-popped popcorn with a hot-air popper.
- When the menu calls for cheese, use a nonfat or reduced-fat option and keep the serving size at ¼ cup or less.
- Use whole-grain tortillas made with only corn, water, and lime.
- Use whole-grain pancake/waffle mix with natural ingredients.
- Instead of using iceberg lettuce (which has almost no nutritional value), use romaine, spring mix, red leaf, green leaf, or other dark green lettuce.
- When a recipe calls for ground beef, use 96 percent fat-free beef.

- When cooking mushrooms, you don't need oil or butter— the flavor comes out all on its own.
- When coating a pan, use extra-virgin olive oil. Put in just a few drops and then wipe the surface with a paper towel so the pan is just barely coated. This will ensure that the food doesn't stick but won't add unnecessary fat to your food.

General Exercise Guidelines

- Make sure that the whole family has good walking/ running shoes that are comfortable and fit properly.
- Keep water nearby when you're exercising so you stay hydrated. At any sporting-goods store, you can buy water bottles that Velcro to a belt around your waist so you don't have to hold your water while you exercise.
- Sign your child up for an active sport five days a week. This could be one sport that meets daily or several sports that meet a few times a week. Give your child input on which sport (or sports) are chosen; the only requirement is that it has to be challenging enough for your child to break a sweat.
- If you can't find an organized sport to join, make up your own activities, such as doing jumping jacks and jumping rope in the backyard, walking up and down the stairs ten times, jumping in an inflatable bounce house, doing crunches and push-ups together, playing Wii Fit, playing soccer with the neighbors, jumping on a trampoline, or going to a dodgeball arena.
- Your goal for walking should be to work up to four miles per hour. It's okay to start slower at the beginning, but you should be getting faster each time.
- On your days off, try to do something fun and active as a family. Go to the park and throw a Frisbee, go to a nearby

lake or river and spend time walking and admiring the outdoors, go ice-skating or roller-skating, or find another active hobby you can enjoy together. This is a good way to instill in your kids that being healthy can be integrated into every part of life while also providing good family bonding time.

• Remember: no excuses!

RECIPES

These are the recipes we used during Breanna's weight-loss journey and beyond. You can, of course, modify them to suit your family's taste. Most of them are very simple and don't require any cooking expertise—I had no idea how to cook healthy foods when I started, but it turned out to be much easier than I anticipated. I've broken these recipes into categories by breakfast, lunch, and dinner, but keep in mind that you can use them interchangeably.

BREAKFAST

Some of these recipes are good for school mornings; others are more time consuming and work great for a weekend. You can make some of them ahead of time, enabling you to quickly heat them in the morning. On school mornings, Breanna often eats one of the following: whole-grain cereal and a small green smoothie, an egg with ketchup and toast, or a single-serving container of fat-free Greek yogurt, fresh fruit, and a piece of dry toast.

Green Smoothie

7 cups fresh spinach
¼ cup nonfat milk or almond milk or soy milk
¼ cup frozen blueberries
½ frozen banana
3 strawberries
1 carrot, peeled
raspberries, blackberries, pineapple, or other fruits, optional

Put the spinach into your blender. (It blends down to very little, so don't worry if it looks like a lot!) Add the milk, blueberries, banana, strawberries, carrot, and any optional ingredients. Blend all ingredients until smooth. Add a bit of milk or water to reach desired consistency.

Yield: 1 adult smoothie, or 2 kid-sized smoothies.

Contains 0 grams of fat.

Simple Scrambled Egg

1 large egg
1 tablespoon milk
½ teaspoon olive oil
1 tablespoon salsa, optional

In a small bowl, beat the egg with the milk until frothy. Heat the olive oil in a nonstick pan over medium heat. Pour egg mixture into the pan, stirring occasionally. Cook until the egg is no longer runny. Top with salsa, if desired.

Yield: 1 serving

Contains 5 grams of fat.

Veggie Omelet

1 egg
splash of nonfat milk, almond milk, or soy milk
fresh herbs of your choice (such as garlic or cilantro)
½ teaspoon olive oil
vegetables of your choice (peppers, mushrooms, asparagus, spinach, broccoli, onions—get creative!), chopped
¼ cup reduced-fat cheese (4.5 grams of fat or less per serving)
1 tablespoon salsa, optional

Whisk together the egg, milk, and herbs. Heat the olive oil in a nonstick pan over medium heat. Pour the egg mixture into the pan; cover. When the egg is just starting to solidify, sprinkle the veggies and half the cheese on top. Cover again and cook until completely solidified. Fold omelet in half and sprinkle with the remaining cheese. Top with salsa, if desired.

    Yield: 1 serving
    Contains 9.5 grams of fat.

Yogurt Parfait

8 ounces nonfat plain Greek yogurt or nonfat honey-flavored Greek yogurt
½ cup fresh fruit of your choice (blueberries, raspberries, strawberries, bananas)
¼ cup low-sugar granola (be careful with granola—it tends to be high in sugar)
ground flax seeds (optional)

Note: The idea is to have a ton of fresh fruit and a small amount of granola.

Layer yogurt with granola and fruit, or just mix it all together. Top with ground flax seeds, if desired.

Yield: 1 serving

Contains 6 grams of fat.

Breakfast Strawberry Sundae

½ cup fresh strawberries

8 ounces nonfat honey-flavored Greek yogurt

1 tablespoon crushed unsalted peanuts, almonds, walnuts, or pecans

1 serving homemade strawberry sauce (see note)

1 fresh cherry

Note: You can make homemade strawberry sauce by combining 1 teaspoon pure maple syrup and 8 strawberries in a blender. Puree until smooth. Yields 4 servings.

We love to serve this pretty breakfast in a sundae glass. Layer strawberries and yogurt; repeat until you're almost at the top of the glass. Pour strawberry sauce and sprinkle crushed peanuts (or other nut of your choice) over the last layer. Top with a cherry.

Yield: 1 serving

Contains 5 grams of fat.

English Muffin with Egg and Bacon

1 whole-grain English muffin

1 scrambled egg (see Simple Scrambled Egg recipe)

½ slice American cheese, or other cheese of your choice

1 slice nitrate-free turkey bacon, cooked

Note: This recipe is great for rushed mornings.

Toast the English muffin. Place cooked scrambled egg on top, followed by cheese and bacon. Microwave for 10 seconds to melt the cheese.

Yield: 1 serving

Contains 8.5 grams of fat

Peachy Cinnamon Bread

1 slice whole-wheat artisan bread, sliced thin
1 peach, cut into thin slices
2 tablespoons nonfat honey-flavored Greek yogurt
Pinch of cinnamon
Honey, for drizzling

Toast the bread. Meanwhile, line a baking sheet with parchment paper. Put the peach slices on the baking sheet and broil just enough to caramelize the sugar. You'll know they are done when the peaches are just slightly soft and starting to brown. They will smell a bit like caramel. Put the peaches on top of the toast, then top with yogurt. Sprinkle with cinnamon and drizzle with a small amount of honey.

Yield: 1 serving

Contains 2 grams of fat.

French Toast

1 egg
¼ cup nonfat milk, almond milk, or soy milk
ground cinnamon
4 slices sprouted whole-grain bread
homemade strawberry sauce (see recipe on p. 260)
2 cups strawberries, sliced

Whisk together egg, milk, and cinnamon. Heat a nonstick pan over medium heat. Dip each slice of bread into the egg mixture and place in pan. Cook until the bottom side is golden brown, then flip and cook the other side. Top with homemade strawberry sauce and sliced strawberries, if desired.

Yield: 4 servings

Contains 3 grams of fat.

LUNCH

Asian Marinade

2 tablespoons low-sodium soy sauce

2 tablespoons honey

2 teaspoons sesame seed oil

¼ teaspoon garlic powder

¼ teaspoon powdered ginger

3 tablespoons pineapple juice

Mix all ingredients together in a small bowl.

Yields enough to marinate four servings of meat.

Contains 2.5 grams of fat per serving.

Turkey Sandwich

2 slices sprouted whole-grain bread

3 slices nitrate-free turkey, ham, pastrami, or chicken

1 slice low-fat Swiss cheese

1 handful romaine lettuce or spinach

Raw vegetables of your choice, such as tomatoes, onions, cucumbers, mushrooms, bean sprouts, or bell pepper, sliced

Layer the meat, cheese, and vegetables between the slices of bread.

Have fun experimenting with different combinations—your child will be surprised how delicious a crunchy cucumber or bell pepper can taste in a sandwich. This is a basic sandwich; you can make substitutions to taste (but no mayonnaise or other high-fat sauces, other than a little bit of mustard).

Yield: 1 serving

Contains 2 grams of fat.

Canadian Bacon Quesadilla

½ teaspoon olive oil
1 tortilla
2 slices 96% fat-free Canadian bacon, cooked
¼ cup low-fat shredded cheese
Vegetables of your choice, chopped

Heat olive oil in a nonstick pan over medium heat. Place tortilla in pan. Add Canadian bacon, cheese, and veggies in the middle of the tortilla. Cover and cook until cheese is melted. Fold in half and enjoy!

Yield: 1 serving

Contains 8.5 grams of fat.

Chicken Quesadilla

1 teaspoon olive oil, divided
1 boneless, skinless chicken breast, cubed into bite-sized pieces
Pinch smoked paprika
Pinch garlic powder, or other salt-free spices or fresh herbs
1 teaspoon lemon juice
1 tortilla

¼ cup low-fat shredded cheese

1 tablespoon diced onion

¼ cup raw spinach

1 tablespoon fat-free sour cream

1 tablespoon salsa

Heat a ½ teaspoon olive oil in a nonstick pan. Put diced chicken in the pan with the paprika, garlic, and other spices of your choice. Stir occasionally. When the chicken is about halfway cooked through, add the lemon juice. Continue stirring until chicken is cooked through (when you cut a piece in half, there should be no pink remaining). Set aside.

In another pan (or wash and reuse your original pan), heat the remaining ½ teaspoon olive oil. Place tortilla in the pan. Add the chicken, cheese, onion, and spinach. Cover and cook until cheese is melted and spinach is tender, then fold in half. Serve with fat-free sour cream and salsa.

Yield: 1 serving

Contains 8.5 grams of fat.

Chef's Salad

2 cups spring mix salad blend

½ hard-boiled egg, sliced

3 slices nitrate-free ham or turkey

red onions, chopped

green onions, chopped

cilantro, chopped

celery, chopped

feta cheese

dried cranberries

cucumbers, sliced

mushrooms, sliced
2 tablespoons low-fat dressing of your choice

Note: Traditionally, a chef's salad includes ham, turkey, hard-boiled eggs, Swiss cheese, American cheese, and bacon, but your goal is to make it healthier. So get creative with your veggies, meats, and legumes! Feta cheese is a good option because it's so flavorful that a little goes a long way. I also like to chop up all the ingredients so you get a mix of flavors in every bite.

Chop the toppings of your choice. Layer spring mix lettuce, egg, meat, and other toppings of your choice. Toss with dressing.

Yield: 1 serving

Contains 8.5 grams of fat.

Garlic Shrimp Tacos

20 large shrimp, peeled and deveined
Juice of ½ lemon
1 tablespoon smoked paprika
1 tablespoon parsley
1 tablespoon minced garlic
8 small tortillas
2 cups chopped romaine lettuce
½ cup cilantro
¼ cup chopped red onions
1 sliced avocado
8 tablespoons salsa
4 tablespoons fat-free sour cream

Heat a nonstick pan over medium-high heat. Add shrimp, lemon juice, smoked paprika, parsley, and garlic to the pan. Cook for 2 to 3 minutes, stirring occasionally, until shrimp are pink and garlic is fragrant. Remove from pan, then cut shrimp into bite-size pieces. Set aside.

In a separate pan (or wash and reuse your original pan), heat 1 teaspoon water over medium heat, and then add two tortillas and cover. Flip after 1 minute, re-cover, and cook until thoroughly heated. Place tortillas on a plate and top with the shrimp, lettuce, cilantro, onion, and avocado. Top each taco with 1 tablespoon of salsa and ½ tablespoon fat-free sour cream.

Yield: 4 servings of 2 tacos each

Contains 7 grams of fat.

Bruschetta

1 small loaf whole-grain artisan bread
1½ cups ripe tomatoes, chopped
6 fresh basil leaves, thinly sliced or chopped
½ cup chopped red onion (optional)
1 tablespoon balsamic vinegar
1 tablespoon olive oil
4 servings fresh mozzarella, thinly sliced
low-fat balsamic glaze

Cut the bread into thin slices. Mix together the tomatoes, basil, red onion (if using), vinegar, and olive oil, and set aside.

Line a baking sheet with aluminum foil and put the bread on the baking sheet. Broil the bread just long enough to make it crispy (it should be golden brown). Remove bread from oven, place a slice of cheese on each piece of bread, and broil again until cheese is bubbly.

Remove from oven and place bread on a plate. Spoon the tomato mixture on top of each slice. Drizzle with balsamic glaze.

Yield: 4 servings

Contains 5 grams of fat per serving.

Bean and Cheese Burrito

4 tortillas
1 (16-ounce) can fat-free refried beans
1 cup reduced-fat shredded cheese
4 tablespoons red onion, chopped (optional)
4 tablespoons salsa

Preheat oven to 450 degrees and line a baking sheet with foil. Heat 1 teaspoon of water in a nonstick pan. Put tortillas in the pan and cover. Cook until heated through. Remove tortillas from pan and place on the baking sheet. Top each tortilla with beans, cheese, onions (if using), and salsa. Fold in half and bake for 5 minutes or until they reach desired crispiness.

Yield: 4 servings
Contains 6 grams of fat per serving.

Asian Chicken Pita

4 whole-grain pitas
3 boneless, skinless chicken breasts, cooked and shredded
2 cups shredded lettuce
4 tablespoons low-fat Asian dressing
1 large carrot, peeled and shredded
20 grapes, halved
1 small handful chow mein noodles

Note: This a great item to pack for a school lunch.

Preheat oven to 400 degrees. Place pitas on a baking sheet and bake until warm. Meanwhile, toss together lettuce, dressing, carrots, and grapes. Remove pitas from oven and cut each in half. Fill pitas with the lettuce mixture and chicken. Sprinkle a few chow mein noodles on top.

Refrigerate any chicken leftovers for another meal.

Yield: 4 servings

Contains 7 grams of fat per serving.

Asian Shrimp Spring Rolls

16 shrimp, peeled and deveined

8 rice-paper sheets

1 bag coleslaw mix (no mayonnaise)

8 tablespoons low-fat Asian dressing

Mandarin oranges, for garnish

In a medium-sized saucepan, bring 2 cups of water to a boil over high heat. Add the shrimp to the boiling water and cook briefly until pink (about 5 minutes). Drain shrimp in a colander, then place shrimp on a cutting board and cut each in half. Set aside.

In a small bowl, mix the Asian dressing with the coleslaw. Set aside.

Cook the rice paper sheets according to the directions on the package and place on a plate. Spoon the coleslaw mixture onto the rice paper. Place 2 shrimp on top of each piece and roll up like a burrito. Cut in half. Serve with mandarin oranges on the side.

Yield: 4 servings

Contains 5 grams of fat per serving.

Chicken, Veggie, and Brown Rice Bowls

4 boneless, skinless chicken breasts

1 serving Asian Marinade (see recipe on page 262)

2 zucchini, sliced thick

1 teaspoon olive oil

2 tablespoons of your favorite herbs and spices (I recommend cilantro, ginger, and garlic for this recipe)
2 cups brown rice, cooked

Put chicken in a plastic bag with the marinade. Refrigerate for 3–4 hours. In a medium-sized bowl, toss zucchini with olive oil and herbs. Thread zucchini onto skewers.

Heat grill on medium-high. Place chicken breasts and zucchini skewers on grill. Flip chicken and zucchini every 2–3 minutes. Continue grilling until chicken is cooked through (no pink remaining when you cut into it) and zucchini is soft but not mushy.

Split the 2 cups of rice among 4 bowls (½ cup rice in each), and top with chicken and zucchini.

Yield: 4 servings

Contains 4.5 grams of fat per serving.

Chicken Salad

4 cups spring mix
20 grapes
2 carrots, peeled and shredded
¼ cup green onion, chopped
1 tomato, chopped
8 tablespoons low-fat salad dressing of your choice
3 boneless, skinless chicken breasts, cooked and shredded
¼ cup feta cheese
4 tablespoons roasted sunflower seeds

In a large salad bowl, toss together spring mix, grapes, carrots, green onion, tomato, and dressing. Add chicken and sprinkle the cheese and sunflower seeds on top.

Yield: 4 servings

Contains 8 grams of fat per serving.

Ham and Swiss Wrap

1 tortilla

2 teaspoons mustard (optional)

2 slices nitrate-free ham

1 slice reduced-fat Swiss cheese

1 large handful shredded cabbage or shredded lettuce

Note: This is a great wrap for school lunches—it can be modified in a variety of ways and has a good balance of nutrients.

Lay tortilla flat and spread with mustard (if using). Layer ham and cheese on top. Add cabbage or lettuce and roll tightly. Cut in half.

Yield: 1 serving

Contains 6 grams of fat.

Make-Your-Own Pizza

For the pizza:

1 teaspoon olive oil

4 pieces lavash bread

1 cup pizza or spaghetti sauce (store bought is fine as long as it's fat free and low in sugar)

1 cup shredded reduced-fat mozzarella cheese

½ teaspoon dried basil

For the toppings:

1 small onion, chopped

1 cup nitrate-free ham, cut into thin strips

Chunks of fresh pineapple

Broccoli, chopped

Tomato, diced

Mushrooms, sliced thin

Olives, sliced

Asparagus, chopped
Corn, cooked
Bell peppers, cut into thin strips

Preheat oven to 425 degrees. Arrange all ingredients on the counter. Drizzle the olive oil onto a large baking sheet and spread with a paper towel, or line the tray with nonstick foil. Arrange lavash on the tray. Spread sauce on top of each piece and sprinkle with cheese and basil. Add as many healthy toppings as you like. Bake until the cheese is bubbly and the bread has reached desired crispiness.

    Yield: 4 servings

    Contains 5–8 grams of fat, depending on the toppings you choose.

Healthy Fried Rice

1 cup scrambled eggs
3 cups brown rice, cooked
1 cup zucchini, chopped
½ cup green onion, chopped
1 cup corn
½ cup carrots, shredded
½ cup bok choy, chopped
½ cup green beans, ends removed
2 tablespoons low-sodium soy sauce
½ teaspoon powdered ginger
2 teaspoons sesame seed oil

Prepare scrambled eggs and rice and set aside. In a wok or nonstick pan, add the rice, zucchini, green onion, corn, carrots, bok choy, green beans, soy sauce, and powdered ginger. Cook over medium-high heat, stirring occasionally, until veggies are tender. Add the scrambled eggs and sesame seed oil. Cook two more minutes until heated through.

Yield: 4 servings

Contains 4 grams of fat per serving.

Asian Chicken Salad

1 bag coleslaw mix (no mayonnaise)

¼ cup sliced almonds

3 green onions, chopped

1 carrot, peeled and shredded

Fresh cilantro, to taste

4 tablespoons low-fat, low-sugar Asian dressing

4 boneless, skinless chicken breasts, cooked and shredded

In a large bowl, toss together the coleslaw mix, almonds, green onions, carrot, cilantro, and dressing. Top with chicken.

Yield: 4 servings

Contains 8 grams of fat per serving.

Make-Your-Own Tacos

1 (1-pound) tri-tip steak, fat trimmed off

1 (15-ounce) jar of salsa

8 tortillas

Toppings of your choice:

2 cups lettuce, shredded

1 small onion, chopped

2 ripe tomatoes, diced

¼ cup fresh cilantro, chopped

¼ cup olives, sliced

¼ cup mushrooms, sliced

1 lemon or lime
4 tablespoons fat-free sour cream (optional)
8 tablespoons salsa (additional, for topping)

Place the steak in a slow cooker and pour the whole jar of salsa over the top. Cook on low for 7–8 hours. Use two forks to shred the meat, and then set aside.

Preheat oven to 400. Line a baking sheet with foil. Place tortillas on the baking sheet and put into oven. Bake until warm.

Arrange the tortillas on a plate. Top with meat and other toppings of your choice. Squeeze the lemon or lime over the tacos for extra flavor. Serve with sour cream and salsa, if desired.

Yield: 4 servings

Contains 6 grams of fat per serving.

DINNER

Grilled Chicken and Veggie Skewers

4 boneless, skinless chicken breasts, cubed into bite-sized pieces
¾ cup marinade, divided (try mixing some lemon juice with smoked paprika and garlic, or use a salad dressing that's low-fat, low-sugar, and free of chemicals)
1 bell pepper, sliced
1 red onion, cut into wedges
1 zucchini, cut into thick slices
1 package white button mushrooms

Put the chicken in a plastic bag or a bowl and pour ½ cup of the marinade over it. Let the chicken marinade in the refrigerator for several hours (or overnight).

Light your grill to medium heat. Thread chicken, peppers, onion, zucchini, and mushrooms onto skewers. Place skewers on grill, rotating them every 5 minutes and brushing with the extra marinade (so they don't dry out). Continue grilling until chicken is cooked through and vegetables are tender (about 20 minutes).

Yield: 4 servings

Contains 4 grams of fat per serving.

Soy Tofu

1 package of tofu
2 tablespoons low-sodium soy sauce
Pinch of nutritional yeast

Heat a nonstick pan over medium heat. Cut tofu into cubes and add to pan. Add soy sauce and sprinkle nutritional yeast on top. Cook, stirring occasionally, until heated through. Serve with veggies on the side.

Yield: 4 servings

Contains 4 grams of fat per serving.

Meat Loaf

1 pound lean ground turkey
1 pound lean ground sirloin
¼ cup whole-grain breadcrumbs
1 egg, beaten
¼ cup onion, chopped
1 tablespoon garlic, minced
1 tablespoon dried thyme
1 tablespoon dried rosemary
½ teaspoon pepper

3 tablespoons Dijon mustard
2 tablespoons milk

Preheat oven to 400 degrees and lightly grease a baking sheet
with olive oil (or line with nonstick foil). Put all ingredients into
a large bowl and mix well. Shape mixture into a loaf and place
on the baking sheet. Bake for 45–55 minutes until a meat ther-
mometer registers 160 degrees. Serve with Mashed Cauliflower
(see recipe on page 287) and Parmesan Spinach (see recipe on
page 286).

   Yield: 8 servings
   Contains 7 grams of fat per serving.

Teriyaki Chicken

4 tablespoons low-fat, low-sugar teriyaki sauce (or make your
own using 4 tablespoons low-sodium soy sauce and 1 teaspoon
sesame seed oil)
½ tablespoon minced garlic
1 teaspoon ginger
1 tablespoon toasted sesame seeds
4 bone-in, skinless chicken breasts

In a small bowl, mix together the teriyaki sauce, garlic, ginger,
and sesame seeds. Pour into a plastic bag. Add chicken; shake
bag until chicken is coated. Refrigerate for 2–3 hours.

   Preheat oven to 375 degrees. Place chicken in a baking dish
and bake for 45 minutes, or until cooked through. Serve with
your favorite veggies.

   Yield: 4 servings
   Contains 5 grams of fat.

Pot Roast in Mushroom Sauce

1 box low-fat cream of mushroom soup (2.5 grams of fat or less per serving; made with natural ingredients)

1 tablespoon dried rosemary

2 tablespoons dried thyme

1 tablespoon minced garlic

4 potatoes, cut in half lengthwise

3½-pound extra-lean beef roast

In a large bowl, mix together cream of mushroom soup, rosemary, thyme, and garlic. Place roast in the bowl and coat with the soup mixture, then place the roast in a slow cooker. Coat potatoes in the soup mixture and then add them to slow cooker. Pour the rest of the mixture on top of the roast. Cook on high for 6 hours.

Serve with your choice of fresh vegetables. (I like to serve this dish with Parmesan Spinach [see recipe on p. 286].) Remember that one serving of meat is the size of your palm, and half the plate should be filled with vegetables. Refrigerate leftovers.

Yield: Serves 8

Contains 7.5 grams of fat per serving.

Ranch Chicken with Corn on the Cob

½ cup low-fat ranch dressing

4 boneless, skinless chicken breasts

4 russet potatoes

4 tablespoons fat-free sour cream

2 ears of corn on the cob

Pour the ranch dressing into a plastic bag. Put the chicken breasts into the bag and shake to coat. Place in the refrigerator for 2 hours.

Preheat the oven to 425 degrees. Wash the potatoes, puncture each several times with a fork, and wrap them in foil. Bake until fork tender, about 45–60 minutes.

While the potatoes are baking, wrap the corn in foil. Light your grill and let it warm up over medium heat. Place chicken and foil-wrapped corn on the grill. Flip chicken and corn occasionally, cooking for about 20 minutes, until chicken is cooked through (no pink remaining) and corn is tender.

Serve chicken with a baked potato, 1 tablespoon of sour cream, and a ½ ear of corn.

Yield: 4 servings

Contains 5 grams of fat per serving.

Nathan's Pork Chops

4 boneless pork chops
4 teaspoons fat-free, all-natural pork rub or seasoning (you can find this in the spice aisle of your grocery store)

Note: This is Nathan's favorite meal, hence its name.

Light your grill and let it warm up over medium heat. Rub each pork chop with 1 teaspoon of the seasoning. Place pork chops on grill, flipping occasionally. Cook the pork chops for 15–20 minutes, depending on how thick they are. Serve with your favorite veggies.

Yield: 4 servings

Contains 8 grams of fat per serving.

Chicken and Mushrooms

4 skinless, bone-in chicken breast halves (6 ounces each)
4 teaspoons Dijon mustard
2 teaspoons of your favorite dried herbs
2 (8-ounce) packages white button mushrooms, sliced

1 tablespoon fresh lemon juice
1 tablespoon fresh parsley, chopped
4 tablespoons shredded Parmesan cheese (optional)

Preheat oven to 375 degrees. Place chicken in baking dish. Brush chicken with mustard; sprinkle with herbs. Top with mushrooms, lemon juice, and parsley. Bake 30–35 minutes, until chicken is cooked through (there should be no pink remaining when you cut into it) and mushrooms are tender. Sprinkle Parmesan cheese on top of each chicken breast, if desired.

Yield: 4 servings

Contains 3 grams of fat per serving.

Grilled Asian Steak

1 pound lean red meat, such as sirloin tip or top sirloin steak
4 tablespoons low-sodium soy sauce
1 teaspoon powdered ginger

Note: Buy the leanest piece of meat you can find.

Wrap steak in plastic wrap or parchment paper. Tenderize the steak by beating it with a meat cleaver, hammer, or rolling pin. Remove plastic or parchment and brush the steak with the soy sauce and sprinkle with powdered ginger.

Heat your grill to high. Grill the steak until cooked to your liking, flipping once (7–10 minutes for medium-rare, 9–12 minutes for medium, and 12–15 minutes for medium-well). Serve with brown rice and a salad.

Yield: 4 servings

Contains 6 grams of fat per serving.

Breanna's Cheeseburgers

4 extra-lean ground beef patties
4 slices reduced-fat Swiss cheese
4 sprouted whole-grain hamburger buns or pitas
1 large tomato, sliced
½ onion, sliced
1 cup romaine lettuce
ketchup, to taste (optional)
mustard, to taste (optional)

Note: This is one of Breanna's favorite meals.

Heat grill on high. Put hamburger patties on grill and cook to your liking, flipping occasionally (6–7 minutes for medium-rare, 7–8 minutes for medium, or 9–10 minutes for well-done).

When burgers are done, place cheese on top. The heat from the burgers will melt the cheese. Serve on buns with tomato, onion, and lettuce. Top with ketchup or mustard, if desired.

Yield: 4 servings

Contains 7 grams of fat per serving.

Cheesy Barbecue Chicken Tortillas

3 boneless, skinless chicken breasts, cubed into bite-sized pieces
1 teaspoon garlic powder
1 teaspoon salt-free seasoning or herbs of your choice
4 whole-grain tortillas
8 tablespoons low-sugar barbecue sauce
¼ cup cilantro, chopped
1 teaspoon onion powder
1 cup reduced-fat cheese
1 cup romaine lettuce, chopped
4 tablespoons salsa

Heat olive oil in a nonstick pan over medium heat. Add the diced chicken, garlic, and other seasoning or herbs of your choice. Stir occasionally until chicken is cooked through. (There should be no pink remaining when you cut into it.) Set aside.

Heat grill on medium. Place each tortilla on a small, individual sheet of aluminum foil. Spread 2 tablespoons barbecue sauce on top of each tortilla. Top with chicken, cilantro, onion powder, and cheese. Grill until cheese is bubbly and tortillas are heated through. Remove from grill, cut into fourths, top with chopped lettuce and salsa, and serve with raw carrots or a side salad. Alternatively, you could heat the tortillas using the same process in your oven heated to 400 degrees.

Yield: 4 servings

Contains 7 grams of fat per serving.

Angel Hair Pasta with Spaghetti Sauce

2 ounces whole-grain angel hair pasta, uncooked
½ cup spaghetti sauce (store-bought, jarred sauce is fine if it is low in sugar)
Vegetables of your choice, chopped (mushrooms, peppers, and onions work well for this dish)

Note: If you cook the whole package of pasta, use 4–6 quarts of water. A single 2-ounce serving of cooked pasta is 1 cup.

Bring 2 cups of water to a boil in a saucepan without any added broth, salt, or butter/oil. Add pasta and cook for 8–9 minutes, stirring occasionally. Meanwhile, heat sauce in microwave or saucepan and add your veggies. Drain the pasta and top with sauce. Simple and delicious!

Yield: 1 serving

Contains 4.5 grams of fat.

Zucchini Pasta

4 zucchini
2 cups spaghetti sauce (store-bought is fine as long as it's low in sugar)
4 tablespoons grated Parmesan cheese
Fresh herbs of your choice, such as basil or parsley

Note: There are multiple devices available for making "pasta" out of vegetables. The simplest to use are probably the spiral peelers. Just wash the zucchini and twist it through the peeler, and it comes out in thin strips that look like cooked spaghetti. You can also use a knife to slice the zucchini into fine strips.

Bring 8 cups of water to a boil in a saucepan. Add the zucchini noodles to the boiling water and stir immediately so they don't stick together. Continue cooking, stirring occasionally, for 3–4 minutes. Drain the zucchini and top with spaghetti sauce, Parmesan cheese, and herbs.

Variation: You can serve this with two medium-sized meatballs made from ground turkey or extra-lean ground beef.

Yield: 4 servings

Contains 3 grams of fat per serving.

Beef Kabobs

1 pound lean red meat, such as sirloin tip or top sirloin steak
4 tablespoons low-sodium soy sauce
1 teaspoon powdered ginger
Vegetables of your choice, cut into chunks (peppers, onions, mushrooms, and zucchini work well for this)

Choose the leanest cut of beef you can find and tenderize it with a mallet or hammer. Rub the soy sauce into the beef and sprinkle it with ginger. Cut the beef into cubes and thread onto skewers, along with the vegetables.

Light your grill on high. Place skewers on the grill and barbecue with the cover closed until the meat is cooked to your liking (about 8–10 minutes). Rotate the skewers several times as they cook. Serve with mashed cauliflower or brown rice.

Yield: 4 servings

Contains 8 grams of fat per serving.

Grilled Honey and Soy Sauce Chicken

4 boneless, skinless chicken breasts
4 tablespoons low-sodium soy sauce
1 tablespoon honey

Marinate chicken with the soy sauce in a plastic bag or in a bowl for 2–3 hours in the refrigerator. Before cooking, brush the top of the chicken with honey.

Light your grill to medium. Barbecue until cooked thoroughly, about 12–15 minutes, flipping chicken several times. Serve with baked cauliflower and steamed spinach.

Yield: 4 servings

Contains 2 grams of fat per serving.

Orange and Honey Baked Chicken

4 boneless, skinless chicken breasts
½ cup orange juice, freshly squeezed
1 teaspoon grated orange peel
4 teaspoons honey

Place chicken in a plastic bag or bowl with the orange juice and orange peel. Let it marinate in the fridge for 2–3 hours.

Preheat oven to 400 degrees. Place chicken in a baking dish and brush with honey. Bake chicken for 30–40 minutes, until juices run clear and there's no pink in the center. Serve with brown rice and veggies.

Yield: 4 servings

Contains 2 grams of fat per serving.

Chicken Nachos

1 teaspoon olive oil
4 boneless, skinless chicken breasts, diced
¼ teaspoon garlic powder
¼ teaspoon paprika
1 teaspoon parsley
8 corn tortillas
1 cup low-fat shredded cheese
2 ripe tomatoes, diced
3 green onions, chopped
¼ cup cilantro, chopped
4 tablespoons fat-free sour cream
4 tablespoons salsa

Preheat oven to 425 degrees. In a nonstick pan, heat olive oil over medium heat. Add the chicken, garlic, paprika, and parsley. Stir occasionally until chicken is cooked through, about 8–10 minutes.

Meanwhile, cut tortillas into eighths. Place tortillas on the baking sheet, and bake to desired crispiness. Arrange tortillas on plates, then sprinkle with cheese. Microwave until melted. Place cooked chicken on top and layer with tomatoes, onions, cilantro, sour cream, and salsa.

Yield: 4 servings

Contains 7 grams of fat per serving.

Potato Kale Soup

1 teaspoon olive oil
1 yellow onion, chopped
1 clove garlic, or ½ teaspoon minced
4 medium-sized red potatoes, diced
5½ cups fat-free chicken broth, divided
1 bunch kale, chopped and steamed
¼ teaspoon rosemary
½ teaspoon thyme
Pinch of black pepper, to taste
4 tablespoons grated Parmesan cheese

In a large pot, heat olive oil and add the chopped onions and garlic. Stir constantly, cooking until onions are tender and translucent, and garlic is fragrant. Add diced potatoes and 3 cups of the chicken broth. Reduce heat and simmer until potatoes are soft, about 15 minutes.

Remove half of the cooked potatoes and puree using a blender. Return the pureed potatoes to the pot. Add the remaining 2 ½ cups chicken broth, kale, rosemary, thyme, and pepper. Heat through. Serve topped with Parmesan cheese.

Yield: 4 servings

Contains 4 grams of fat per serving.

SNACKS AND SIDES

Tomato, Basil, and Mozzarella Salad

1 large tomato, sliced
2 fresh basil leaves, thinly sliced
1 ounce fresh mozzarella cheese (about the size of a Ping-Pong ball), sliced
1 teaspoon balsamic vinegar glaze

Layer the tomato slices, basil, and cheese. Drizzle with balsamic vinegar glaze.

Yield: 1 serving

Contains 4.5 grams of fat.

Baked Zucchini

¼ cup panko whole-wheat bread crumbs
1 zucchini
All-natural, salt-free seasoning of your choice (garlic powder, lemon pepper, or dried cilantro would work well)

Preheat oven to 450 degrees and line a baking sheet with foil. Quarter the zucchini so it's in four long, thin pieces. Place bread crumbs in a shallow dish. Press zucchini slices into the bread crumbs (firmly, so that the bread crumbs stick). Lay the zucchini on the baking sheet and bake for 10 minutes. Sprinkle with seasoning.

Yield: 1 serving

Contains 1.5 grams of fat per serving.

Slow Cooker Applesauce

5 pounds apples, peeled, cored, and thinly sliced (any variety is fine, but Honeycrisp apples are exceptionally good)
1 ½ tablespoons ground cinnamon
½ teaspoon ground cloves
¼ teaspoon ground nutmeg

Layer apples in a slow cooker and sprinkle cinnamon, cloves, and nutmeg over the top. Cook on high for 4–5 hours. You can whisk the apples by hand or use a potato masher for chunky applesauce. Or, puree the apples with an immersion blender or in an upright blender for smooth applesauce. You can store leftovers in the refrigerator for up to a week, or you can freeze them for up to 6 months.

Yield: 16 servings

Contains 0 grams of fat per serving.

Baked Cauliflower

1 head cauliflower

1 tablespoon salt-free seasoning of your choice (garlic powder and rosemary work well for this)

¼ cup grated Parmesan cheese

Preheat oven to 400 degrees, and line a baking sheet with foil. Cut cauliflower into bite-sized pieces, place on the baking sheet, and sprinkle with seasoning. Sprinkle with Parmesan cheese and 2 tablespoons of water, and cover loosely with aluminum foil. Bake for 15 minutes, then remove the foil and bake for another 5 minutes for added crispiness.

Yield: 4 servings

Contains 4 grams of fat per serving.

Parmesan Spinach

3 cups raw spinach

1 tablespoon grated Parmesan cheese

Heat a nonstick pan over medium heat. Place raw spinach in the pan with a few drops of water. Stir constantly until spinach is wilted. Sprinkle with Parmesan cheese. How easy is that?

Yield: 1 serving

Contains 1 gram of fat per serving.

Healthy Cauliflower "Mashed Potatoes"

1 teaspoon garlic powder
1 teaspoon all-natural, salt-free seasoning of your choice
1 head cauliflower

Note: If this is too big of a leap from mashed potatoes, transition by replacing half of your potatoes with mashed cauliflower.

Cut cauliflower into several pieces. Steam or boil until soft, about 8–10 minutes. Pour into a bowl, add garlic and other seasoning, and mash with a potato masher.

Yield: 4 servings

Contains 0 grams of fat.

No-Fry French Fries

4 potatoes, any variety
1 tablespoon all-natural, salt-free seasoning of your choice
2 teaspoons olive oil

Preheat oven to 425 degrees. Peel and rinse potatoes. Cut into thin, French fry–like slices. Pat potatoes dry with a paper towel. In a large mixing bowl, toss together the potatoes, olive oil, and your seasoning of choice. Place French fries on a baking sheet and bake until crispy and golden-brown, about 35–40 minutes, turning potatoes occasionally. Serve with organic ketchup (it doesn't contain high-fructose corn syrup like conventional ketchup does).

Yield: 4 servings

Contains 2 grams of fat per serving.

Hummus

1 (15.5-ounce) can garbanzo beans, drained
1 tablespoon lemon juice
2 tablespoons tahini
1 teaspoon cumin
½ teaspoon garlic powder

Note: This recipe makes a base hummus that is great on its own, but you can also experiment by adding other vegetables. Have fun figuring out how to make hummus that's both healthy and tasty.

Blend all ingredients in a food processor. Serve with strips of red pepper or carrots.

Yield: 4 servings

Contains 2.5 grams of fat per serving.

Oven-Baked Chips

4 corn tortillas
2 spritzes olive oil spray

Preheat oven to 425 degrees. Cut tortillas into eighths. Place on baking sheet. Spray with olive oil spray. Bake to desired crispiness, about 7–10 minutes. Serve with hummus or guacamole.

Yield: 4 servings

Contains 2 grams of fat per serving.

Collard Green Chips

10 collard green leaves
1 teaspoon lemon juice
1 teaspoon Parmesan cheese, grated

Note: For this recipe, you'll need a food dehydrator. This is an investment, but it can come in handy. You can make far more than collard green chips with it—you can also make any kind of veggie chips, homemade fruit leathers, or homemade jerky.

Chop the collard greens into bite-sized pieces and put them into a plastic bag. Add lemon juice and cheese, close the bag tightly, and shake. When everything is well mixed, put the collard greens into the dehydrator. Cooking time will vary based on the model—be sure to read the instructions and check for doneness.

Yield: 1 serving

Contains 1 gram of fat per serving.

Guacamole

1 avocado, peeled
¼ cup salsa
¼ teaspoon garlic powder

Mash avocado in a bowl. Mix in the salsa and garlic powder. Serve with carrots or homemade tortilla chips.

Yield: 4 servings

Contains 3 grams of fat per serving.

Blueberry "Ice Cream"

2 frozen bananas
¼ cup fresh blueberries
¼ cup milk

Blend banana, blueberries, and milk in a blender until smooth and creamy, about 2–3 minutes. Done—it is that easy.

Yield: 1 serving

Contains 0 grams of fat per serving.

Pineapple Delight

¾ cup frozen pineapple chunks
2 tablespoons nonfat milk, almond milk, or soy milk

Put pineapple and milk into blender. Blend until smooth. Enjoy!
 Yield: 1 serving
 Contains 0 grams of fat per serving.

Strawberry Ice Pops

2 frozen bananas
½ cup fresh strawberries

Blend banana and strawberries together in a blender. Leave at room temperature until the mixture becomes liquid, then pour into ice pop molds. Place in freezer for several hours, until frozen through.
 Yield: 4 ice pops
 Contains 0 grams of fat per serving.

Pineapple-Blueberry Freeze

¼ cup frozen pineapple chunks
¼ cup fresh blueberries

Blend the pineapple chunks and blueberries together in a blender and enjoy. Delicious!
 Yield: 1 serving
 Contains 0 grams of fat per serving.

SHOPPING LIST

Note: This is a general list of staples rather than an exhaustive grocery list.

Grains

    whole-grain tortillas

    sprouted whole-grain or flaxseed bread

    quinoa

    brown rice

    brown rice pasta

    oatmeal (preferably steel-cut)

    whole-grain cereal

    low-sugar granola

    popcorn kernels

    rice cakes

    whole-grain pitas

    whole-grain English muffins

    whole-grain buns

    whole-grain wraps

Produce

vegetables (all kinds—try things you've never tried before!)
various kinds of lettuce for salads
fruits (strawberries, raspberries, blueberries, bananas, apples, oranges)
dates coated in oat flour (as an occasional treat)
raisins
fresh herbs of your choice

Dairy

fat-free milk
eggs
nonfat Greek yogurt (plain and honey flavored)
fat-free sour cream
reduced-fat shredded cheese
feta cheese
Parmesan cheese
fresh mozzarella
low-fat or nonfat cottage cheese

Protein

extra-lean ground beef (96 percent fat-free)
lean red meat, such as sirloin tip or top sirloin steak
nitrate-free turkey, ham, pastrami, or chicken
extra-lean ground turkey (96 percent fat-free)
turkey bacon (nitrate-free)
tofu
pork
beef jerky (nitrate-free)
beans of all kinds (fat-free refried beans, lentils, pinto beans, split peas)

powdered peanut butter
raw nuts (almonds, cashews, pecans)

Condiments and Spices

hummus
Dijon mustard
salsa
salt-free seasoning
powdered cinnamon
dried rosemary
dried thyme
dried dill
white pepper
black pepper
onion powder
garlic powder
organic ketchup
smoked paprika
paprika
tarragon
pork rub
poultry rub
steak rub
bay leaves
chili powder
dried oregano
dried sage
nutritional yeast
salt-free Italian seasoning
ground ginger
ground turmeric

ground marjoram
mint
curry powder
Chinese five-spice powder
dried parsley
ground coriander
low-fat/fat-free dressings
low-sodium soy sauce
all-natural barbecue sauce

Miscellaneous

extra-virgin olive oil
reduced-sodium chicken broth
chickpeas
low-sugar orange juice
olive oil spray
low-fat balsamic dressing
honey
pure maple syrup
spaghetti sauce
lemon juice

Frozen Foods

frozen strawberries (not in syrup)
frozen blueberries (not in syrup)
frozen raspberries (not in syrup)
frozen shrimp (deveined)
flash-frozen fish
flash-frozen chicken breasts (not breaded or in
    a marinade)

Q&A WITH BREANNA

Q: How is your life now different than it was a few years ago?

A: I wasn't in sports before, and now I love sports! Life is so much better when you can do the things you love. I also don't get teased anymore. If you are overweight, you probably know what I'm talking about. It was the same routine every day: wake up, go to school, get made fun of at recess and lunch, and then go home and hide in my room and cry and ask God to fix me. Now I have way more friends, and I'm happier too—just more excited about things.

Q: What was the hardest part of your journey to becoming healthier?

A: The hardest part was when I first started. Walking was so hard then—I just wasn't used to it, and it was hard for me to keep up. But the more I worked at it, the easier it got. After I walked for a while, I started running, and now I can't believe I'm actually sprinting! It was really hard at first, but it gradually got easier.

Q: What is the best part of being healthy?

A: I started water polo this year, and I absolutely love it! I never could have done that a couple of years ago. I was also really excited when I found out I was one of the few people who qualified for a big swimming competition, which is coming up in a few months. The top ten from each division qualified, and I can't believe I was one of them.

Q: What do you like to do in your free time?

A [laughing]: I don't really have much free time! Between water polo, swimming, cheerleading, doing homework, spending time with my family, and hanging out with my friends, I don't really have time for much else.

Q: How has your perspective on food changed in recent years?

A: I eat completely differently now. And surprisingly, I actually like the foods my mom makes, even though I didn't at first. Another big change is that back then I was always thinking about food, wondering what the next meal or snack would be and when I'd get to eat. But now I just don't care as much— I have so many other things I'm thinking about.

Q: What advice would you give to other kids who are struggling with their weight?

A: I would tell them, "Never give up, no matter how hard it is. I've been through this, and if I can do it, I know you can too. It will get easier, I promise." I would also say, "Don't wait! Now is the time to get healthy so you can live life to the fullest and enjoy what God has in store for you."

Q: How did your parents help you on this journey?

A: They set goals for me and encouraged me all along the way. If you are a parent, keep pushing your kid. They'll say, "You're so mean" and "You're torturing me," but don't give up. It will be worth it in the end.

Q: How has your faith helped you on this journey to becoming healthy?

A: There were definitely tough times along the way—times when I felt depressed and sad or like I couldn't keep going. But I prayed to God in those times, and he gave me the strength I needed to make it. Whenever you feel down, just remember that you can do all things through Christ who gives you strength!

AFTERWORD

This was a challenging but rewarding journey for us, and Breanna and I are happy to have the chance to encourage others along the way. I hope this book has been helpful for you, and I hope you see the same dramatic results we have.

If there's anything I can do to help you on your path, or if you just want to reach out and say hello, please contact me through Breanna's website, www.breannabond.com, or on Facebook at https://www.facebook.com/breannabond online. That's where we'll continue to share updates about what Breanna is up to, and we'd love to post your success story too.

Thank you for reading our story. We wish you all the best as you embark on your life-changing journey to health.

ACKNOWLEDGMENTS

I want to acknowledge Breanna for the courage and strength it took not only to overcome childhood obesity but also to share her journey with the world. Breanna, through you, others will know that change is possible. You are opening people's eyes, hearts, and minds to the reality of this epidemic that is hurting one-third of children in the United States and countless others throughout the world. By having the courage to share the struggles and insights from your journey, you are empowering others who are fighting the same battle we did and leading the way for them to take a stand and create change in their lives. I am so proud of you.

I would also like to acknowledge Kerry Nichols, my mentor and friend, for giving me a voice when I did not have one. Thank you for the countless hours you sacrificed to make this book happen. It could never have happened without you.

Special thanks to my literary agent, Ruth Samsel, at William K. Jensen Literary Agency for all the hard work you have put into this project. Thank you for your counsel, guidance, support, and belief in me throughout the process of writing this book. It has been such a pleasure working with you.

I would also like to thank everyone at Tyndale House Publishers for all the months of work it took to make this book a reality, with special thanks to Carol Traver, Stephanie Rische, Stephen Vosloo, and Jackie Nuñez.

Above all, I would like to thank my writer and friend Jenna Glatzer for all the hours you put into writing this book. You are one of the best, most sought-after writers in America, and I am truly blessed to have you. You are also one of the sweetest, most compassionate people I have ever had the privilege of knowing. It has been an honor working with you, and I'll miss our late-night conversations.

A special thanks to CNN, *The Biggest Loser*, *Good Morning America*, and *The Today Show* in Australia for sharing Breanna's story with the world.

Nathan, I am so proud of you for being such a sport when our lives seem so chaotic at times. You are a trooper and a champ, and I am forever grateful. I love you always.

And thank you, Dan, for being my rock and my best friend. I could not have gone through this journey without your love and support. I love you.

Notes

1. JoAnn Stevelos, "Bullying, Bullycide and Childhood Obesity," Obesity Action Coalition, http://www.obesityaction.org/educational-resources /resource-articles-2/childhood-obesity-resource-articles/bullying-bullycide -and-childhood-obesity.
2. Barbara Pinto, "Was a 10-Year-Old Honor Student Bullied to Death?" ABC News, November 15, 2011, http://abcnews.go.com/blogs /headlines/2011/11/was-a-10-year-old-honor-student-bullied-to-death/.
3. Jessica Hopper, "Suicide Pact: Minnesota Teens Haylee Fentress and Paige Moravetz Commit Suicide at Slumber Party," ABC News, April 20, 2011, http://abcnews.go.com/US/suicide-pact-minnesota -eighth-graders-haylee-fentress-paige/story?id=13411751.
4. Jotham Suez, et al., "Artificial Sweeteners Induce Glucose Intolerance by Altering the Gut Microbiota," Nature 514 (October 9, 2014): 181–186.
5. http://www.aacap.org/AACAP/Families_and_Youth/Facts_for_Families /Facts_for_Families_Pages/The_Depressed_Child_04.aspx.
6. Michael Moss, "The Extraordinary Science of Addictive Junk Food," New York Times, February 20, 2013, http://www.nytimes.com /2013/02/24/magazine/the-extraordinary-science-of-junk-food .html?pagewanted=all&_r=0.
7. "Warning Signs of Bullying," Mayo Clinic, August 23, 2013, http://www.mayoclinic.org/healthy-living/childrens-health/in-depth

/bullying/art-20044918?pg=2. See also Joel Haber, *Bullyproof Your Child for Life* (New York: Penguin, 2007).

8. "Warning Signs of Bullying," Mayo Clinic, August 23, 2013, http://www.mayoclinic.org/healthy-living/childrens-health/in-depth /bullying/art-20044918?pg=2.

9. L. Murtagh and D. Ludwig, "State Intervention in Life-Threatening Childhood Obesity," *Journal of the American Medical Association* 306, no. 2 (July 13, 2011): 206.

10. "Physical Activity Guidelines for Americans," President's Council on Fitness, Sports, & Nutrition, http://www.fitness.gov/be-active/physical -activity-guidelines-for-americans/.

11. Mark Hyman, "Sweet Poison: How Sugar, Not Cocaine, Is One of the Most Addictive and Dangerous Substances," *New York Daily News*, February 10, 2014, http://www.nydailynews.com/life-style /health/white-poison-danger-sugar-beat-article-1.1605232.

12. J. Wilson, "Girl Loses 65 Pounds in Fight against Childhood Obesity," CNN, July 21, 2014.